VEGAN ONE-POT WONDERS

To Jude, my lover of food.
Thank you for trying and
loving every single recipe
in this book. You make
the world a better place.

This book was created
on the traditional land
of the Wurundjeri People.

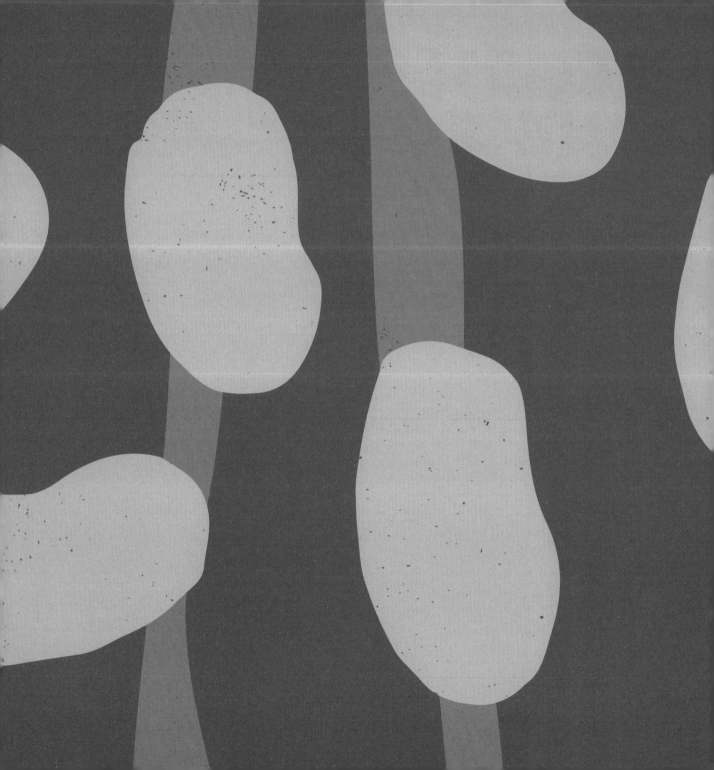

VEGAN ONE-POT WONDERS

Easy, delicious, plant-based meals for the modern home cook

JESSICA PRESCOTT

PHOTOGRAPHY BY
BEC HUDSON

Hardie Grant
BOOKS

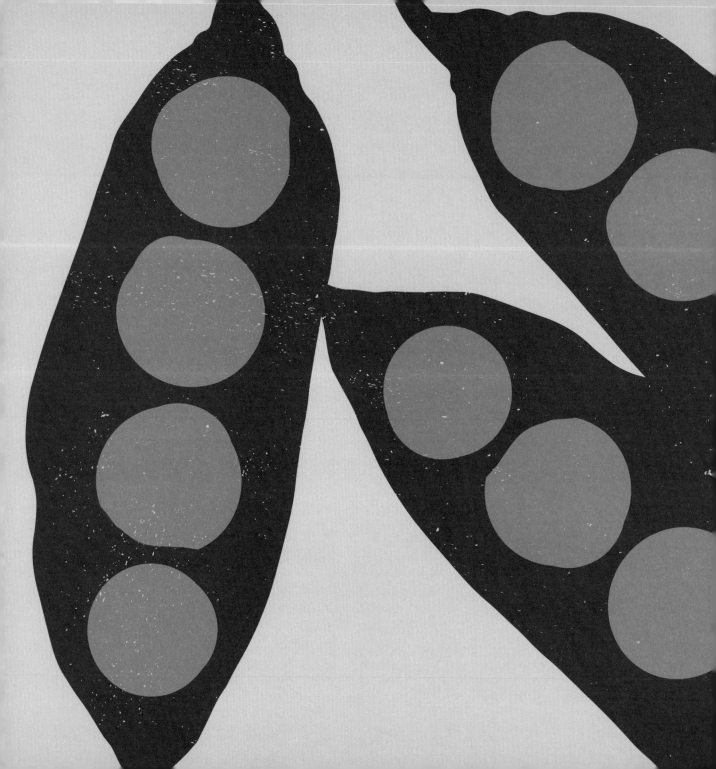

Preface

There's no doubt about it, 2020 has been a strange year.

When I sat down to write the introduction of this book in January, it was with a fervor caused by the fact that the country I call home was ablaze. I wondered if the 2020's would be named the Roaring Twenties for a different reason this time, after the fires and floods that defined the turn of the decade, leaving in their wake an unimaginable amount of heartache, suffering and loss.

Fast forward to April, and we are in the midst of another unprecedented crisis – COVID-19. Much of the world is in lockdown, with those who have the privilege to do so distancing ourselves from one another in an attempt to slow the growth of this catastrophic pandemic.

No one knows how long our new way of living will go on, or what life will be like when it's over, but dealing with this on the heels of the climate catastrophe has many of us riddled with helplessness, despair, and increasing anxiety in the face of so much uncertainty.

As we tighten our purse strings and brace ourselves for a global recession, now more than ever it's important to remember that our future is quite literally in our hands. Every time we spend money we are casting a vote for the type of world we want to live in, and moving forward, this must look different. Buying less. Supporting small, ethical companies. Changing to banks that don't invest in fossil fuels, weapons and animal agriculture. Using our cars less. Saying no to single use plastics. These are all achievable changes that collectively, send a clear message.

If we are really passionate about the future of our species (because let's face it, Mama Earth will be just fine without us) we must change what we put on our plates. How this looks will differ from person to person, but in order to maintain the dietary requirements of our growing population and make the most efficient use of our precious land and water in the least impactful way, we need to take the focus away from meat and dairy. Animal agriculture is one of the major contributors to climate change and the exploitation of animals is thought to be the cause of all of the new and major pandemics we have faced in the last 40 years.

It's a wretched time, but there are pockets of beauty; one silver lining is that home cooking is making comeback. I hope that this book will fill your homes with delicious, effortless and inexpensive meals that nourish your body and soul while being kind to the planet.

Thank you for being on this journey with me.

Love Jess xxx
April 2020, Melbourne, Australia

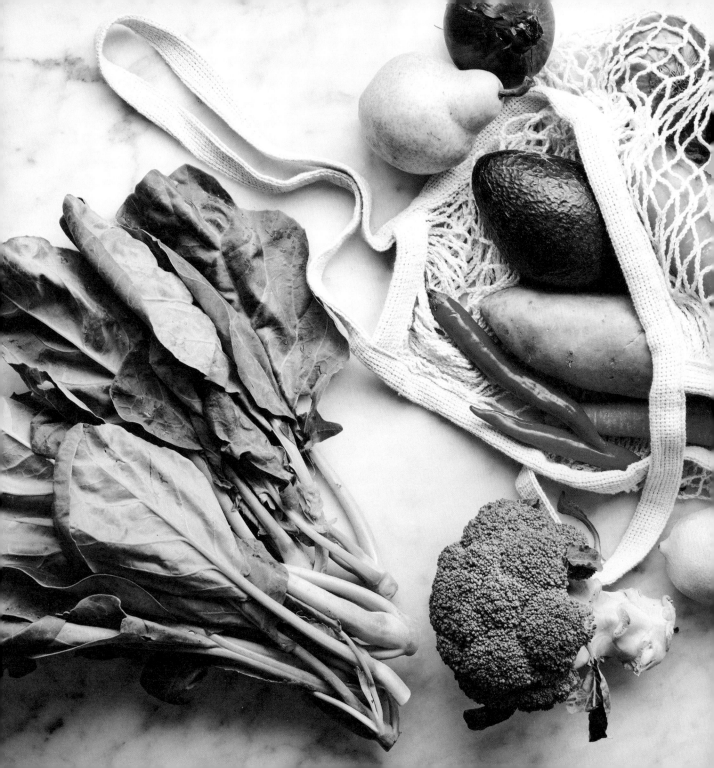

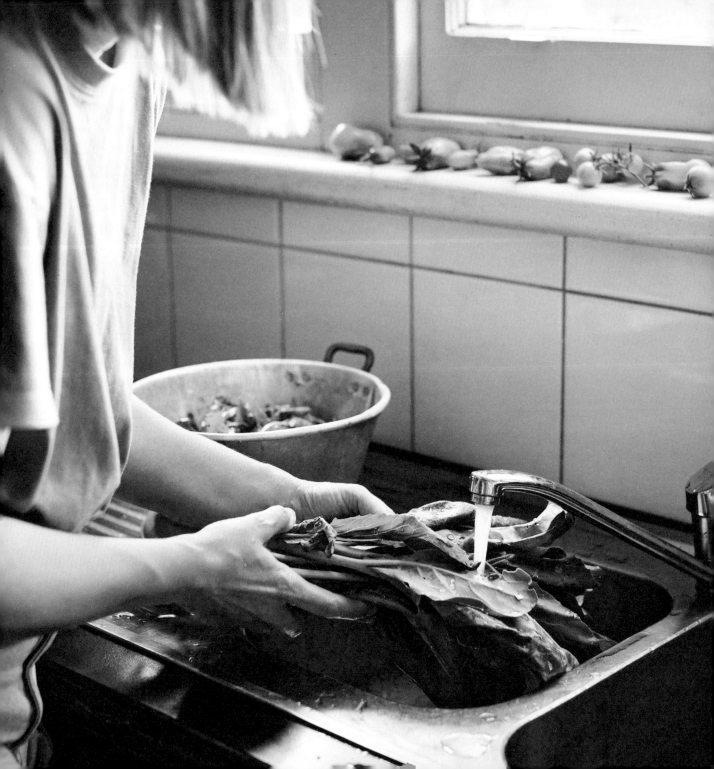

What is a One-Pot Wonder?

I don't know about you, but I'm tired of doing the dishes. Breakfast, lunch, dinner, and if you have small children, a million and one snacks in between. The mess is relentless, which is why I wrote this book. I know I'm not alone when I say I need recipes that nourish the body and soul, while simultaneously being low mess, versatile and easy to prep ahead of time, and kind to the planet.

My first cookbook was a mostly-wholefoods-based vegan 101-style cookbook – the type of book that teaches you new ways to use things you already have in your pantry. My second was a book about feasting, to celebrate and immortalise the many dinner parties my husband Andy and I had on the floor of our Berlin apartment before we had kids, and the way in which sharing food changed once we were parents.

My third cookbook, this one you hold in your hands right now, is for busy people.

A one-pot wonder is a meal where all components are cooked in one vessel, meaning there is only one annoying thing to wash once mealtime is over. There might also be a bowl for rinsing greens or mixing dressing, a colander for draining soaked beans, or some other things that just need a quick rinse or wipe, but only one dish where elbow grease might be required to remove the food.

This type of cooking is essential for me, because I honestly feel like all I do is wash dishes and pick up toys from our floor. All. Day. Long. Over and over again. On repeat. The last thing I need is dinners where I dirty two pots, a pan and a roasting dish. That kind of cooking is okay for when I'm in a cooking mood, but now that I have kids, I need quick, easy and minimal-mess recipes for day to day cooking; things that go just as well with a slice of bread as they do with a side of rice or quinoa.

Almost everything in this book can be served in a multitude of different ways, because I am sure that, like me, you have weeks where you feel like a domestic goddess and weeks where you feel like you are chasing your own tail. Thank goodness for nutritious bread and tinned beans on those weeks.

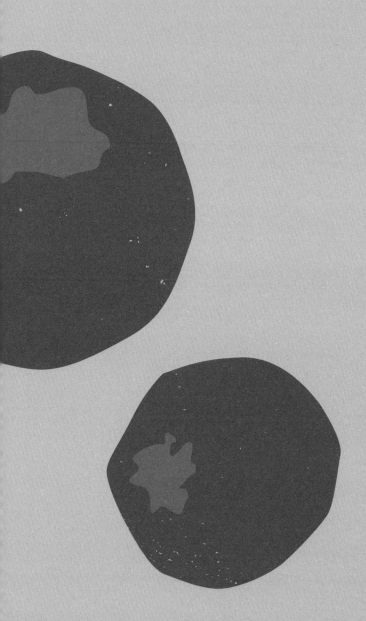

Basics

In this chapter you will find tips and tricks to make the day to day easier, as well as recipes for things that you can make or buy, depending on how you are faring on any particular week.

Pantry Essentials

I've always had a soft spot for a fancy ingredient. It gets harder to splurge on such things when you have multiple mouths to feed, but I do believe in buying the best quality you can afford. This may look different from week to week – it certainly does for us – but at any given time, you will find a combination of the following foods in my pantry.

PROTEINS:

Seeing as this is one of the main things that piques peoples inner nutritionist when they hear my family doesn't eat meat or meat products, I thought I should share some of my top protein sources. Because I am not qualified to dish out nutritional information I don't feel comfortable sharing any in this book, but I recommend to anyone who wants to get an idea of their dietary intake to download the Cronometer app. I don't use it every day, but I do use it to see how balanced my meals are and find it incredibly helpful.

Legumes – I use a lot of beans and lentils in this book, in particular black beans, white beans, chickpeas (garbanzos) and French green (Puy) lentils. I eat them every day and while I try to cook them from scratch, I would be utterly lost without the tinned versions, which I go through many of every week.

Quinoa – an excellent protein source and a great thing to have on hand to bulk up a meal or reinvent leftovers. See page 19 for info on cooking and storing.

Peanut butter – I love all nut butters, but peanut is definitely my favourite and the one I cook with the most. We go through multiple jars a week in my home and you will notice I use it in a few of my recipes. The peanut butter I use contains roasted peanuts and salt. That's it. No sugar and absolutely no palm oil or any other type of oil. It should be runny and pourable and preferably come in a glass jar.

Tofu and tempeh – both are made from soy beans, but, unlike tofu, tempeh is made from the whole bean and also fermented. They are excellent sources of protein, and have the ability to take on the flavours of whatever you are cooking them in. Tofu usually needs to be drained and then wrapped in a clean, lint-free tea towel and placed under something heavy for at least 30 minutes. This gets all of the excess water out and makes room for the flavours to get in.

OTHER ESSENTIALS:

Nutritional yeast – a mainstay in any vegan pantry, this deserves a special mention for anyone who is new to the world of vegan cooking. It is a source of B vitamins and is often enriched with B12 which is the only essential nutrient not available in plant foods. I use it to add an umami element to spice mixes (page 27) for things like scrambled tofu and roasted potatoes as well as sprinkling it straight onto my kids' pasta.

Tinned tomatoes and passata – essential for many of the recipes in this book, I always have a tin, jar or carton of each on hand.

Dried herbs and spices – if nothing else, I will always have various different salts, black pepper, chilli flakes, cumin (whole and ground), coriander (whole and ground), sweet smoked paprika, turmeric, onion powder, garlic powder and nutmeg in my pantry.

Stock – I have a combination of liquid, powdered, bouillon and homemade stocks in my kitchen at all times. Which one I reach for depends on my mood. You can use whatever type you have to hand in most of the recipes in this book where I use stock. Liquid stock is great and always so flavourful, but powdered and bouillon are cheaper and come with less packaging. Homemade is great, but not always as convenient as the stuff you buy in stores. Use what you can. Experiment with different brands until you find ones that you love and check the small print as often the ones that say chicken-'style' and beef-'style' are actually vegan. If you can't find them, use veggie stock in place of chicken, and mushroom stock in place of beef.

Fresh herbs – I am blessed with a decent herb garden in my back yard, which includes rosemary, sage, oregano, parsley, lemon thyme, bay leaf, kaffir lime, basil, Thai basil, mint and Vietnamese mint. If you have the space I highly recommend buying plants of the herbs you use most, as it saves so much money and waste, and is sometimes the difference between needing to duck out to the shops or not when you want to cook a meal.

Bread – this book contains a lot of bread, I know. Having wholesome sourdough bread in my home is essential for me and the way I cook, and making sourdough from scratch is one of the most rewarding tasks you can ever set out to do. I highly recommend finding a starter and looking at the tutorials I have saved on my Instagram (I filmed it when COVID-19 Isolation began and hundreds of people have had incredible success), finding a local sourdough-making course or digging into some cookbooks and learning how to make your own. If you are allergic to gluten, we are lucky to live in a time where delicious gluten-free bread is easily available and there are a kazillion recipes online and in books so that you too can have your own delicious and nutritious bread on hand at all times.

Mock meat – to people who are not vegan or vegetarian, and even to some who are, the idea of mock meat can seem baffling. 'Why not just eat the real thing?' is a question I am often faced with. There are many reasons why, but the main one is that a lot of people who eschew animal products still like the way they taste. Others, like me, get bored of the same protein sources and are curious to see what alternatives are available these days. Either way, there are so many delicious alternatives out there. Some odd ones, too. Try what's available and see how you go, and if all else fails, try the Tofurky brand Italian sausages. They are widely available and so delicious. Processed, yes, but no more than a traditional sausage.

Really good-quality vegan cheese – in Australia – as well as most countries, I'm sure – there are gourmet vegan cheeses of the soft and hard variety that are outrageously delicious. There are also a number of really terrible ones. If you are new to vegan cooking, ask around, see what cheeses vegan restaurants in your city are using, try them all, and you WILL find something you like (if not, stay hopeful). We are so lucky to live in a time where we have innovative people dedicating their lives to bringing us dairy alternatives and while vegan cheeses will never taste like the 'real thing', your tastebuds will adjust.

Dried mushrooms – an excellent way to add flavour to a dish, I use them in a few recipes in this book, soaking them in water first to make a mushroom stock and then chopping up the reconstituted mushrooms to add flavour and texture. Shiitakes are great in Asian dishes and porcini or wild mushrooms are good in everything else.

SOME OTHER NOTES:
I use **tamari** in all of my Asian-inspired recipes because I prefer its light taste compared to soy sauce, but you can swap it for soy sauce if that's all you have.

Most of my recipes call for 3–5 cloves of **garlic**. This is because some cloves are very big and others very small. Three large or 5 small should do it.

Cooking Equipment

In contrast to the pantry list, my kitchen equipment list is pretty minimal. There are definitely a couple of unnecessary things that have crept into my pantry (hello waffle iron, that I swore was going to be my solution to Louie's fussy eating, and the deep-fat fryer we were given two years ago that has never been used), but we don't have the space or money for excess cookware and gadgets, so the things that constitute 'one-pot' in this book are as follows:

- large pot
- medium pot
- small pot
- casserole pot (Dutch oven) that can go in the oven
- frying pan (skillet)
- ovenproof frying pan (skillet)
- baking dish with high sides
- baking tray (sheet pan) with low sides
- blender
- mixing bowl

In addition to these I have glass and plastic jugs of varying sizes, few chopping boards, good knives, mixing bowls, wooden spoons, a grater, a lemon press, a Microplane grater, a mandoline and a non-aerosol olive oil spray (a godsend) all of which I use in this book. The last three are handy but not make-or-break when it comes to cooking any of my recipes. I also own a microwave which I avoided my entire adult life until we were given one when we moved to Melbourne. It has been a total game changer. You can bake a potato in 10 minutes. I mean, enough said!

RECIPE KEY

 Blender

 Mixing bowl

 Frying pan (skillet)

 Saucepan

 Casserole pot

 Baking tray (sheet pan)

 Loaf pan

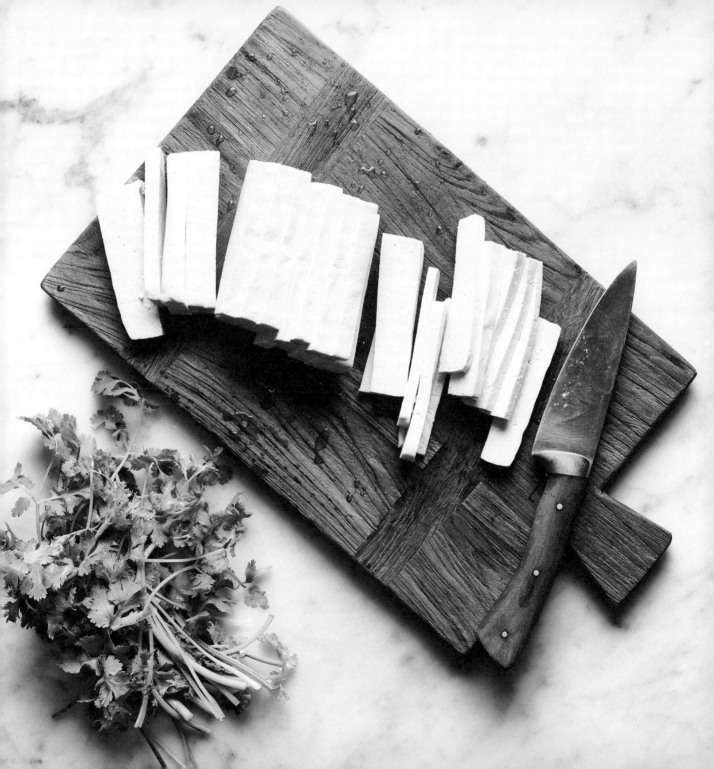

How I cook and other tips for busy people

HAVING A NICE TIME IN THE KITCHEN

I love cooking but it can easily become a chore rather than a peaceful and joyful part of your day when you have small children or an insane work schedule. When you can, clean and tidy your workspace, and gather all of your equipment and ingredients, before you start cooking. I find that the 5–10 minutes spent doing this makes such a difference to my state of being while I am in the kitchen. If you are able to, use your time in the kitchen as time to practise being present. When I cook with intention, I find cooking to be a deeply relaxing and satisfying process. I love listening to music as I go about my day, and especially when cooking, but I also love to cook in silence sometimes, just me and my veggies, having a nice time as I peel and chop and sizzle and stir and appreciate the privilege of being able to create delicious and wholesome meals whenever I want to.

TIME-SAVING/PANTRY MEALS

I find it handy to have a couple of meals in my repertoire that require no fresh ingredients at all. In my case, we always have the ingredients for nachos (page 120), enchiladas (sans salsa on top) (page 131) and socca (page 148), so that if all else fails, we will be fed. I've marked recipes that fit this brief with a 'pantry ingredients only' symbol. Recipes that have minimal chopping and take less prep-time have been marked with a knife symbol so you can see at a glance what should work under a time restraint.

FRIDGE ONE, FREEZE ONE

There is something very rewarding about cooking something that will sustain you over more than one mealtime. I came up with a little method in my early postpartum days with my son Jude, and named it, 'fridge one, freeze one'. The idea is that if I make enough of whatever meal I am cooking for three nights' worth of dinner, I can put some in the refrigerator for later in the week and some in the freezer for later that month. By doing this, you can reduce the time you spend in the kitchen and still have nutritious and warming meals at the beep of a microwave button. Not all of the recipes in this book will make enough food for you to be able to do that, but when you do find yourself with leftovers, most of them will last up to **4 days in the refrigerator and up to 3 months in the freezer**. (Except salad. Salad shouldn't go in the freezer.)

RECIPE KEY

 Pantry ingredients only

 Minimal or no chopping

 Freezes well

 Contains nuts

BAKED POTATOES

Baked potatoes and sweet potatoes are a great way to turn leftover stews and curries into a nutritious, filling and effortless second dinner.

I 'bake' my potatoes in the microwave these days, as it's quicker and therefore more energy efficient. It also means you can enjoy them on a hot day, without making your home even hotter by turning the oven on.

To bake potatoes in the microwave, scrub the skins clean, dry them thoroughly, then poke holes all over the potato either with a fork or a paring knife. Place on a heatproof bowl or plate and microwave for 5 minutes per potato, turning once during cooking time (use tongs for this). Check with a fork: if you cannot easily pierce the potato, continue to microwave at 1 minute increments until it is fork-tender.

Alternatively, you can cook or even finish them off in a hot oven. To do this, preheat the fan oven to 180°C (350°F/gas 6). Wash and dry your potatoes and prick with holes as above, then coat them with olive oil. Place in the hot oven for 1–1½ hours until fork-tender. If you are just finishing them off in a hot oven to get the skin crispy, a good coating of oil (use a brush or spray so you don't burn your hands) and 10 minutes baking should do it.

TOASTING AND ROASTING NUTS AND SEEDS

Toasting or roasting nuts and seeds ahead of time is an excellent way to bring delicious crunch and flavour to your meals. You can do this either in a dry frying pan (skillet) or in the oven. I use both methods, depending on what I am toasting, my mood and the quantity I'm toasting (a baking tray has more room than a frying pan).

Frying pan method: place up to a cup of seeds or nuts in a dry frying pan over a medium heat. Toss frequently for 5–10 minutes until fragrant and starting to change colour. Remove from the heat.

Oven method: preheat the oven to 160°C (320°F/gas 4). Spread up to 2 cups of nuts onto a baking tray and place in the oven for 5–10 minutes, keeping a good eye and nose on them as they can go from okay to burnt in mere seconds (we've all been there with pine nuts haven't we?).

With both methods, you can either allow them to cool in the pan/on the tray, where they will continue to deepen in colour from the heat of the pan/tray, or transfer to a plate and allow to cool there. Once cool, transfer to a clean, dry glass jar where they will stay fresh for up to a month.

If you can get into the habit of almost always having *something* toasted on hand, you'll thank yourself when you use them.

NB: I buy my sesame seeds and peanuts already roasted.

POT PIES

The simple act of laying puff pastry over the top of a stew, then placing it in a hot oven, can turn a stew into a seriously moreish and deeply satisfying meal; comfort food at its finest.

To turn your stew into a pie, you want to cook your stew in an ovenproof frying pan (skillet) rather than a large pot, so that your filling comes almost to the top of the dish. If the thought of this makes you nervous you can use a deeper oven-safe pot. There will be space between the filling and the pastry, but it will be no less delicious.

Lay a sheet or two of puff pastry over the top of your stew, prick with holes, and place in a hot oven for 10 minutes or until the pastry is puffy and golden.

Vegan pastry is pretty easy to find these days; however, finding pastry without palm oil can prove tricky. Palm oil is a monocrop that is responsible for deforestation of rainforests and therefore loss of habitat for many animals, including orangutans, so depending on the reason you have chosen to adopt a vegan diet, you may wish to avoid it.

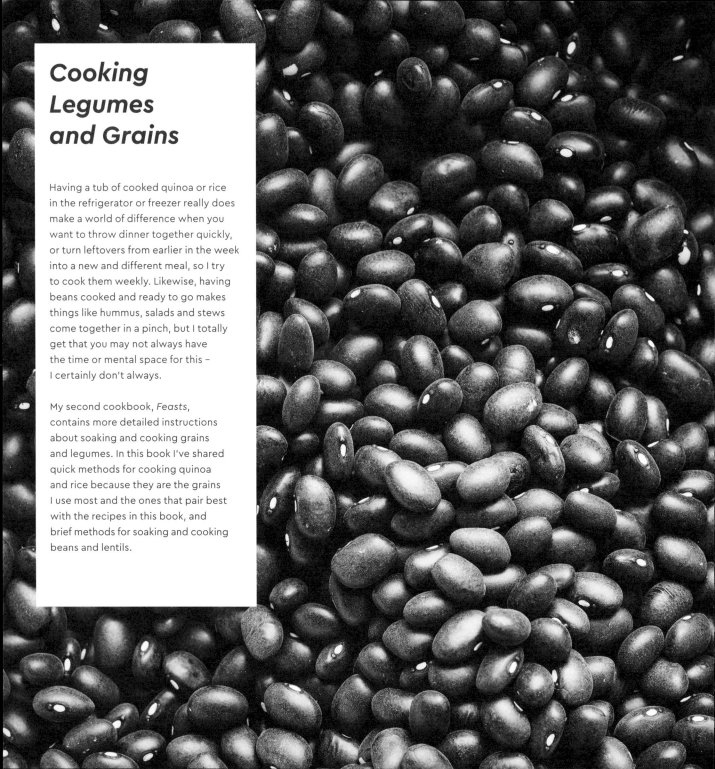

Cooking Legumes and Grains

Having a tub of cooked quinoa or rice in the refrigerator or freezer really does make a world of difference when you want to throw dinner together quickly, or turn leftovers from earlier in the week into a new and different meal, so I try to cook them weekly. Likewise, having beans cooked and ready to go makes things like hummus, salads and stews come together in a pinch, but I totally get that you may not always have the time or mental space for this – I certainly don't always.

My second cookbook, *Feasts*, contains more detailed instructions about soaking and cooking grains and legumes. In this book I've shared quick methods for cooking quinoa and rice because they are the grains I use most and the ones that pair best with the recipes in this book, and brief methods for soaking and cooking beans and lentils.

HOW TO COOK QUINOA AND RICE

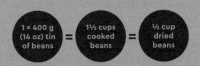

HOW TO COOK BEANS AND LENTILS

Quinoa

Rinse 1 cup of quinoa under cold running water in a fine mesh sieve (strainer) until the water runs clear. Place in a small saucepan with 2 cups of water and ½ teaspoon of salt. Stir, then cover with a lid. Bring to the boil then lower the heat and simmer, covered, for 20 minutes. **Do not remove the lid or disturb it while it is cooking.** Once cooked, remove from the heat and allow to sit for 5–10 minutes. Remove the lid, add a light drizzle of olive oil and fluff the grains with a fork. Allow to sit, uncovered, for 10 minutes. Enjoy immediately with any soup, stew, curry or salad, or cool and store in an airtight container in the refrigerator for up to 4 days or in the freezer for up to 3 months.

Rice

The method for cooking rice is much the same, however white rice will take about 20 minutes to cook and brown rice will take about 40 minutes to cook. If you want to check that all of the water is absorbed, use the handle of a spoon to pull back some of the grains and see if there is still water in the pan, rather than stirring them.

All of the recipes in this book are written with the above ratios in mind, so you can interchange home-cooked and shop-bought with ease.

If you do wish to cook dried beans (including chickpeas/garbanzos) and lentils from scratch, it is beneficial to soak them, both to reduce their cooking time and their nutrient-blocking phytic acid. You will notice that in some of the bean recipes in this book I add bicarbonate of soda (baking soda) to their soaking water. This helps them to break down and cook more quickly, however if you want them to retain their shape, you should skip this step. I use French green (Puy) lentils for almost every lentil recipe in this book; however, you can also use beluga and get the same result. Bicarbonate of soda (baking soda) isn't necessary when soaking and cooking lentils.

Cooking dried beans

Soak 1 cup of beans in a bowl or pan of water with a teaspoon of bicarbonate of soda (baking soda) overnight. Drain and rinse well, then place in a large pot with 1 litre (34 fl oz/4 cups) of water. Cover, bring to the boil, then reduce the heat and simmer for 1–2 hours, checking the softness of the beans every 30 minutes or so by squishing them on the side of the pot. When they start to soften, add a teaspoon of salt and continue to cook until tender (the total amount of time they take will depend on how old and dry they are). Drain.

Cooking dried lentils

Soak 1 cup of lentils in a bowl or pan of water overnight. Drain and rinse, then place in a large pot with 1 litre (34 fl oz/ 4 cups) of water. Cover, bring to the boil, add a teaspoon of salt, then reduce the heat and simmer for 15–20 minutes. After 15 minutes they should be cooked but still have some bite to them. After 20 minutes they should be cooked and soft. Drain.

Cooked beans and lentils can be stored in their cooking water in an airtight container for up to a week in the refrigerator, or 3 months in the freezer. Simply drain off the cooking liquid before using and you are good to go (I rinse tinned beans but don't feel the need with home-cooked ones; however, feel free to do so if you prefer).

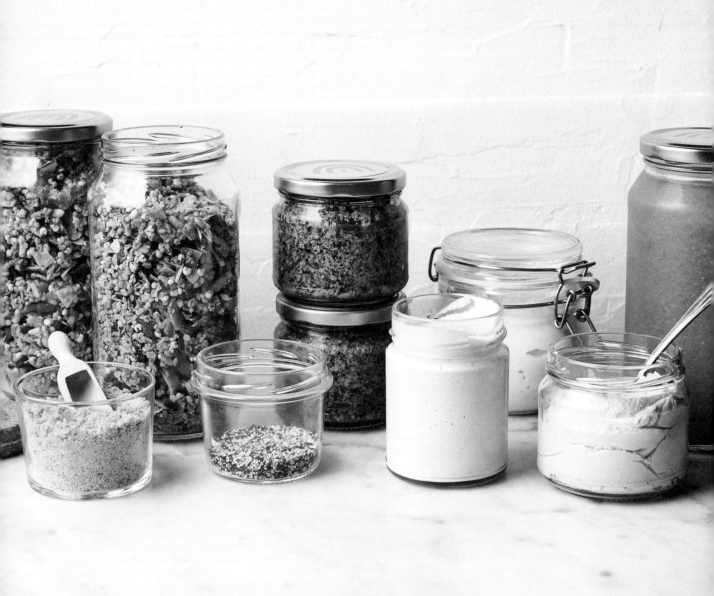

Things You Can Make or Buy

A Green Pesto for Every Season

We always have a jar of pesto in our refrigerator or pantry for bang together meals that could benefit from a dollop or five of something green and oily.

Use this as a master method and sub in any different herbs or nuts you have in excess. I have never used lettuce or chard but I hear it is a great way to use them up if they are beginning to wilt. A favourite at the time of writing this book is kale pesto with toasted almonds. It is truly heaven.

MAKES ABOUT 500 G (1 LB 2 OZ)

1 firmly packed cup of herbs or leafy greens (around 30 g/1 oz)
120 ml (4 fl oz/½ cup) olive oil
60 ml (2 fl oz/¼ cup) lemon juice
½ teaspoon salt
2 garlic cloves, crushed
2 tablespoons nutritional yeast (optional)
45 g (1¾ oz/½ cup) flaked (sliced) almonds, toasted

Put all the ingredients, except the nuts, in a high-speed blender and blend until smooth. Add the nuts and pulse until combined but still a little chunky.

Seasonal variations:
Winter pesto – rosemary, sage, parsley, oregano, lemon thyme, walnuts
Spring pesto – rocket (arugula), basil, pine nuts
Summer pesto – basil, coriander (cilantro), cashews
Autumn (fall) pesto – kale, toasted flaked (sliced) almonds

Butter Bean Hummus

Butter (lima) beans are a delicious alternative to chickpeas (garbanzos) that result in a rich and creamy hummus but by all means, use chickpeas if you prefer. I use unhulled tahini as the flavour really is so much better, but hulled works just fine if that's all you have.

MAKES 500 G (1 LB 2 OZ)

400 g (14 oz) tin of butter (lima) beans, drained and rinsed
100 g (3½ oz/⅓ cup) unhulled tahini
juice of ½ lemon
2½ tablespoons olive oil
½ teaspoon ground cumin
½ teaspoon ground coriander
½ teaspoon salt
1–2 garlic cloves, crushed (minced)
about 60 ml (2 fl oz/¼ cup) cold water

Put all the hummus ingredients in a high-speed blender and blend until smooth. Add more water if you need to – the amount of water you need will depend on how juicy your lemon is. You may need to turn the machine off, remove the lid and scrape down the sides a few times with a spatula to get everything nicely blended.

Use immediately or transfer to an airtight container and store in the refrigerator for up to a week.

Enjoy with bread or organic corn chips, fritters, or even loaded onto a baked potato. Yum!

Goji Goodness Granola

This is my favourite granola recipe. Use it as a guide, keeping basic ratios the same and you wont be disappointed.

I like to serve mine with fresh fruit (usually berries, sometimes banana too), a splash of milk and a dollop of coconut yoghurt. A good friend uses puréed apple as an alternative to yoghurt, which is a tip that definitely needs to be shared with the world.

**MAKES 2 X 1-LITRE
(34 OZ/4½ CUP) JARS**

75 ml (2½ fl oz/⅓ cup) melted coconut oil
150 g (5 oz/⅖ cup) rice malt syrup
150 g (5 oz/1⅔ cup) rolled oats
110 g (3½ oz/1½ cup) puffed rice, puffed quinoa, puffed millet or a combination of all 3
80 g (3 oz/generous 1 cup) flaked coconut
40 g (1½ oz/generous ½ cup) flaked (sliced) almonds
2 tablespoons pumpkin seeds
1 tablespoon chia seeds
1 tablespoon hemp seeds
1 tablespoon flax seeds
1 teaspoon ground cinnamon
1 teaspoon vanilla extract
pinch of salt
generous handful each of goji berries and chopped dried apple, or any other dried fruit

Preheat the oven to 120°C (250°F/gas 1) and line two baking trays (sheets) with baking paper.

Combine the oil and syrup in a large bowl. Add all the remaining ingredients, except the dried fruit, and stir so that everything is well combined and nicely coated with the oily, syrupy concoction.

Spread the mixture out on the baking trays and bake in the oven for 25–30 minutes, giving it a stir about halfway through so that the bits on the outside go into the middle and the bits in the middle go to the outside, until evenly golden.

Remove from the oven and allow to cool on the trays. Break any large chunks into smaller pieces then add the dried fruit before transferring to airtight containers. The granola will keep for a good month or so.

Cashew Cream

A lot of my recipes call for the addition of 'something creamy' at the very end, right before serving. In an ideal world, this will almost always translate to cashew cream. I have spoken of my love for cashews in my previous books; however, for those who don't (yet) own them, I wanted to include a quick recipe for cashew cream and a few ideas on other things you could use instead.

MAKES 400 G (14 OZ)

155 g (5½ oz/1¼ cup) raw cashews
250 ml (8½ fl oz/1 cup) cold water
salt

Soak the cashews in a bowl of salted water overnight or for at least 6–8 hours, or cook them in a saucepan of boiling water for 15 minutes. Drain and rinse under cold running water, then put them in a high-speed blender with the cup of fresh water. Blend until fully incorporated and silky smooth. Use immediately or store in the refrigerator in an airtight container for up to 1 week.

TIP: If all of this is too much for you, fear not. We live in a world with dairy alternatives galore and I find it handy to grab a tub of vegan cream cheese or sour cream every now and again, to have on hand for meals that call for it. Soy and coconut yoghurt also work a treat, just be sure to use a plain (not sweetened) one if using on savoury meals.

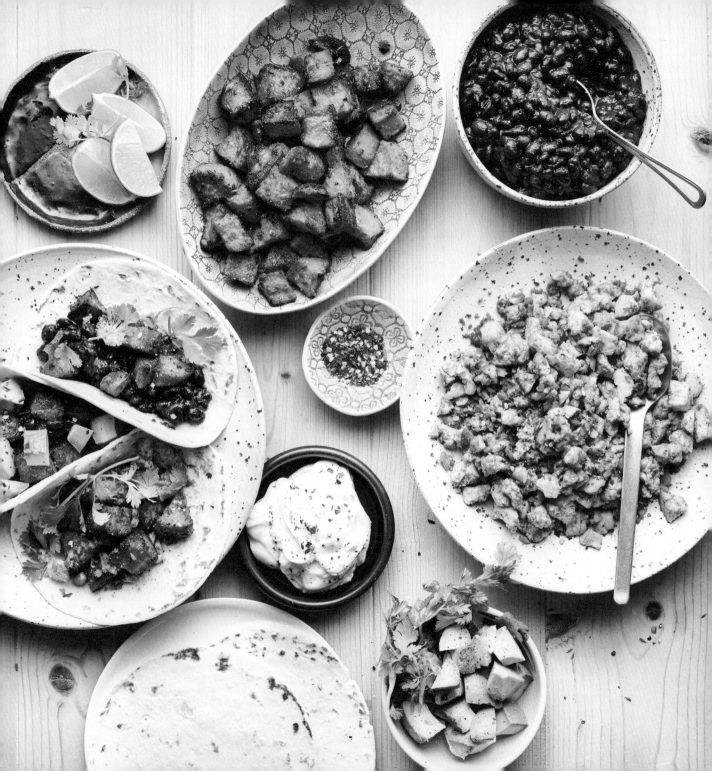

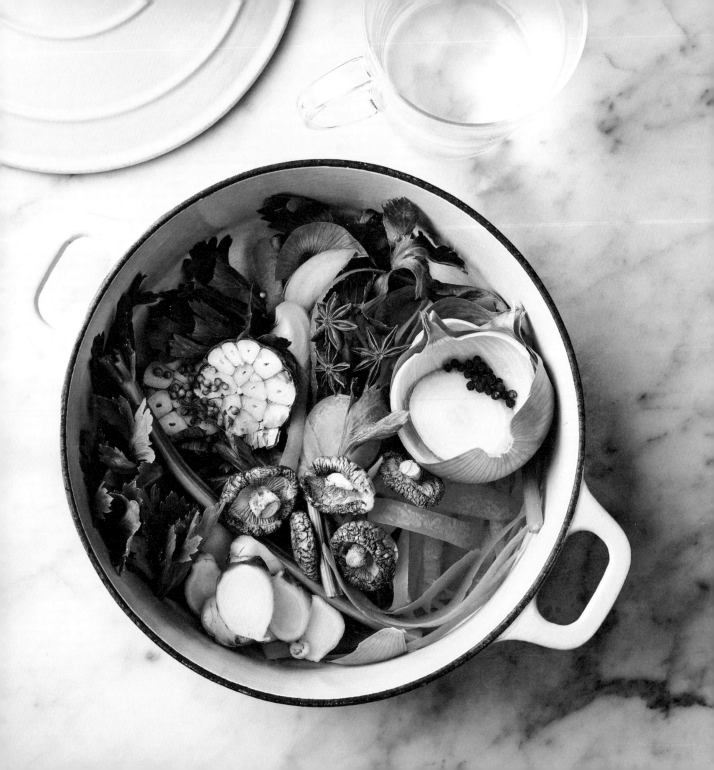

Veggie Scrap Broth

Making your own broth is a great thing to do if you wish to cut cooking costs. Not only can you use peels, skins and root-ends of your veggies, you can also use many veggies lurking in the bottom of your veggie bin that you would otherwise discard – hello floppy carrots, rogue pieces of celery and spring onions (scallions).

It does take time and foresight, which is why I have an array of powdered, liquid and homemade stocks in my pantry at any given time, but there is so much satisfaction in collecting your veggie scraps and then giving them a new life. I encourage you to try it, even if it's not something you do every week.

I like to put my broth-friendly scraps in a large plastic tub in the freezer, until I am ready to give them their second life.

Avoid using the following:
brassicas (broccoli, cauliflower, Brussels sprouts, kale), as they can impart bitterness
vegetables you wouldn't usually cook, such as cucumber and avocado
vegetables that are mouldy, slimy or really dirty

MAKES 3 LITRES (5.2 PINTS/ 12½ CUPS)

skins and root-ends from 3 onions
skins and tops from 3 carrots
root-ends and leaves from 3 celery stalks
1½ teaspoons salt
4 litres (140 fl oz/16 cups) water

Optional extras:
For an Asian-inspired broth
thumb-size piece of fresh ginger, sliced
whole head of garlic, cut in half
10 g (½ oz) dried seaweed (I use wakame or kelp)
5–6 dried shiitake mushrooms (about 10 g/½ oz)
1 tablespoon white peppercorns
5 or 6 Chinese red dates (jujube)
1 tablespoon goji berries
1 lemongrass stalk, halved lengthways
stalks from a bunch of coriander (cilantro)
1 cinnamon stick
3 star anise
1 tablespoon coriander seeds
1 tablespoon white peppercorns

For a Mediterranean-inspired broth
whole head of garlic, cut in half
10 g (½ oz) dried porcini mushrooms
1 tablespoon black peppercorns
discarded tops and bottoms of 1–2 leeks, rinsed well
peels and root-ends from sweet potato, parsnip, or another root vegetable
3 dried bay leaves
leftover herbs such as thyme, rosemary, parsley, or herbs of choice

Put the vegetable scraps in a large stock pot with the salt and any other optional extras, cover with water, bring to the boil, then reduce the heat and simmer, covered, for a couple of hours (skimming scum off the top if necessary). Remove from the heat and leave to cool.

Once cool, strain through a sieve (fine mesh strainer) into another large pot or bowl, squeezing out any extra liquid from the veggies as you do so, before ladling into jars.

Use the stock immediately, store it in a glass jar in the refrigerator for up to a week, or freeze it for up to 3 months. If freezing, don't fill your container all the way to the top, and freeze with the lid loose until the contents are fully frozen before screwing the lid on tightly, as the broth will expand as it's freezing and will crack the glass if it has nowhere to go.

Spice Mixes and Flavour Boosters

These are things I like to prepare in batches, so that when it comes to scrambling some tofu or building a salad, I have everything ready to go. It's little things like this that makes tasty meals come together extra quickly. I don't always have these on hand, but if I have to make up a spice blend for a meal, I make more so that the next few meals come together more quickly. The amount I make usually depends on what size jar I have at my disposal. Be sure to label it – your brain will thank you later.

Salad Topper

4 tablespoons flaked (sliced) almonds
4 tablespoons pumpkin seeds
4 tablespoons sunflower seeds
1 tablespoon cumin seeds

Place all the ingredients in a large, dry frying pan (skillet) over a medium heat and toast for 5–10 minutes, stirring frequently, until golden and fragrant. Allow to cool (in the pan is fine, unless you have let them take on quite a bit of colour, in which case transfer to a plate – if they stay in the pan they'll darken further). Transfer to a clean, dry glass jar and use on top of any salad for a crunch, flavour and nutrition boost.

Sesame Seaweed Salt Blend

There is a company in Australia who makes an umeboshi furikake and it is to die for. It is almost always sold out, so I often throw together my own bootleg version. Seaweed is a source of iodine, which is an essential nutrient that can be difficult to find in plant foods.

4 tablespoons toasted black sesame seeds
4 tablespoons toasted white sesame seeds
4 tablespoons seaweed flakes
4 tablespoons salt flakes

Place all the ingredients in a mortar and pestle and lightly pound, so that seeds are a little broken but still intact. Transfer to a clean, dry glass jar. Sprinkle on top of rice dishes, on fries and popcorn, avocado toast, etc.

Sprinkles

This alternative to Parmesan tastes nothing at all like Parmesan but it hits the spot nonetheless when a dish needs a bit of a boost. I like it on plain spaghetti with olive oil, dried chilli flakes and nothing else, but it is also excellent on top of lasagne and other dishes.

You can make this with walnuts, almonds, cashews and pine nuts, or any combination of the four. Don't stress about the final weight too much. So long as you have about a cup, you'll be fine.

about 100 g (3½ oz/1 cup) toasted nuts of choice
4 heaped tablespoons nutritional yeast
1 teaspoon salt
1 teaspoon garlic powder

Lightly toast the nuts in a dry frying pan (skillet) over a medium heat for 5–10 minutes, stirring frequently to prevent burning, then transfer to a plate and allow to cool. Place in a food processor with the nutritional yeast, salt and garlic powder and pulse until the mixture resembles fine breadcrumbs. Store in an airtight jar until ready to use. It will keep for a good couple of months.

Really Good Potato Seasoning

	FOR ONE RECIPE	FOR THREE RECIPES	FOR SIX RECIPES
onion powder	1 teaspoon	1 tablespoon	2 tablespoons
garlic powder	1 teaspoon	1 tablespoon	2 tablespoons
ground cumin	1 teaspoon	1 tablespoon	2 tablespoons
ground coriander	1 teaspoon	1 tablespoon	2 tablespoons
smoked paprika	1 teaspoon	1 tablespoon	2 tablespoons
sea salt	1 teaspoon	1 tablespoon	2 tablespoons
nutritional yeast	1 tablespoon	3 tablespoons	6 tablespoons

Place all the ingredients in a clean, dry glass jar and stir to combine or put the lid on the jar and turn the jar around so that the contents get evenly distributed. Use 3 tablespoons per 1.2 kg (2 lb 11 oz) potatoes.

Scrambled Tofu Seasoning

	FOR ONE RECIPE	FOR THREE RECIPES	FOR SIX RECIPES
onion powder	1 teaspoon	1 tablespoon	2 tablespoons
garlic powder	1 teaspoon	1 tablespoon	2 tablespoons
ground coriander	1 teaspoon	1 tablespoon	2 tablespoons
smoked or sweet paprika	1 teaspoon	1 tablespoon	2 tablespoons
ground turmeric	1 teaspoon	1 tablespoon	2 tablespoons
black salt	1 teaspoon	1 tablespoon	2 tablespoons
nutritional yeast	2 tablespoons	6 tablespoons	12 tablespoons

Place all the ingredients in a clean, dry glass jar and stir to combine or put the lid on the jar and turn the jar around so that the contents get evenly distributed. Use about 4 tablespoons per 500 g (1 lb 2 oz) tofu.

Mama Goodness Spice Blend

	FOR ONE RECIPE	FOR THREE RECIPES	FOR SIX RECIPES
dried basil	1 teaspoon	1 tablespoon	2 tablespoons
dried oregano	1 teaspoon	1 tablespoon	2 tablespoons
celery seed	1 teaspoon	1 tablespoon	2 tablespoons
sweet or smoked paprika	1 teaspoon	1 tablespoon	2 tablespoons
fennel seeds	1 teaspoon	1 tablespoon	2 tablespoons
dried thyme	1 teaspoon	1 tablespoon	2 tablespoons

Place all the ingredients in a clean, dry glass jar and stir to combine or put the lid on the jar and turn the jar around so that the contents get evenly distributed. Use 2 tablespoons in a pot of spaghetti Bolognese, etc.

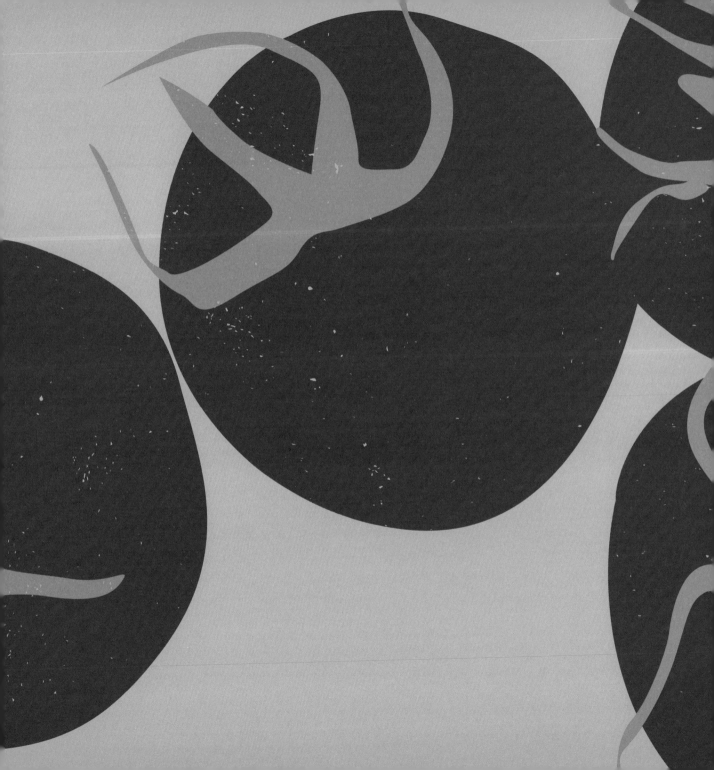

No-Cook Meals

In this chapter you'll find some of my favourite things to bang together when it's too hot to cook.

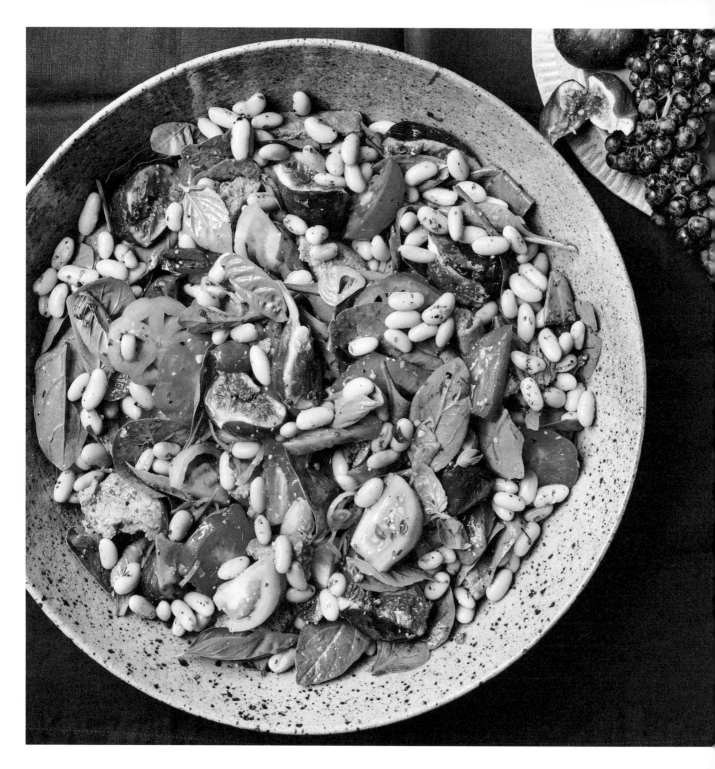

INGREDIENTS

about 600 g (1 lb 5 oz) tomatoes,
    cut into bite-size pieces
about 100 g (3½ oz) olives, halved
    if you can be bothered
400 g (14 oz) tin cannellini (white)
    beans, drained and rinsed
100 g (3½ oz) rusks, crushed
    (see Tip)
about 60 g (2 oz) baby spinach
about 30 g (1 oz) fresh basil leaves,
    torn into bite-size pieces
4–5 fresh figs, torn in half
    (optional)

For the dressing:

120 ml (4 fl oz/½ cup) olive oil
juice of 1 lemon
2 tablespoons sherry vinegar
1 generous teaspoon dried
    oregano
½ teaspoon sea salt
½ teaspoon dried chilli (hot
    pepper) flakes (optional)
1 teaspoon wholegrain mustard
1 tablespoon capers (baby
    capers), finely chopped
    (minced)
1 garlic clove, crushed (minced)
1 large or 2 small shallots, very
    thinly sliced
freshly ground black pepper,
    to taste

End of Summer Rusk Salad

Rusk salad is one of my favourite Greek foods and this version includes marinated beans to make it a meal rather than a side. I make it at the end of summer, when tomatoes and figs are in abundance and it's too hot to cook. I prepare everything in the morning and then it comes together in a pinch when we are ready to eat.

1   Combine the dressing ingredients in a large mixing bowl. Add the tomatoes, olives and beans and stir to well combine. Cover with a dinner plate and allow to sit for at least 30 minutes, stirring every now and then if you remember.

2   When ready to serve, add the crushed rusks and stir so they are well coated in the dressing and tomato juices. Add the spinach, basil and figs (if using). Toss gently and serve immediately.

TIP: If you have stale bread at home that you would like to use in place of rusks, tear it into pieces, coat with olive oil and bake for 10 minutes in an oven preheated to 160°C (320°F/gas 2) until crispy and beginning to turn golden.

SERVES 2–3
(depending on which
toppings you choose)

INGREDIENTS
For the açai:
100 g (3½ oz) block frozen açai
1 frozen banana (see Tip)
115 g (3¾ oz/¾ cup) frozen
    blueberries
90 g (3¼ oz/¾ cup) frozen
    raspberries
250 ml (8½ fl oz/1 cup) coconut
    water, plus extra if needed

For the topping
(as much as you like of each):
granola
fresh fruit
dried fruit
nut butter
nuts
seeds
cacao nibs

Andy's Açai Bowls

Ah-sigh-ee is a berry with a cult superfood status because of its super-high antioxidant levels. Despite the growing popularity of açai bowls over the past few years, I never understood the hype until the fruit store next to my husband Andy's work started selling them and we both got hooked. Now, they are our favourite breakfast or lunch on a hot summer day.

You can use frozen and freeze-dried açai interchangeably. If you use freeze-dried, increase the berries to one cup each and use a tablespoon of freeze dried açai powder.

1   Put all the açai bowl ingredients in a high-speed blender and blend until smooth. You will need to turn the machine off, remove the lid and scrape down the sides a few times with a spatula to get everything evenly and smoothly blended. Add more coconut water to get things moving if you need to.

2   Pop some granola or fruit in the bottom of your serving bowls, if using. Spoon the açai mixture into the bowls, then add whichever toppings you fancy: you can be as minimalist or as decadent as you like. I always add at least a blob of peanut or pumpkin seed butter, and sometimes granola. If I am making this for Andy or a friend I load them up with extra toppings such as fruit, cacao nibs and hemp seeds as well.

TIP: Bananas should be covered in spots before you freeze them. This changes their composition and makes them more fluffy as opposed to gooey when you blend them. Once ready to freeze, peel, break in half and place in a freezer-safe container (in the freezer) until you are ready to use.

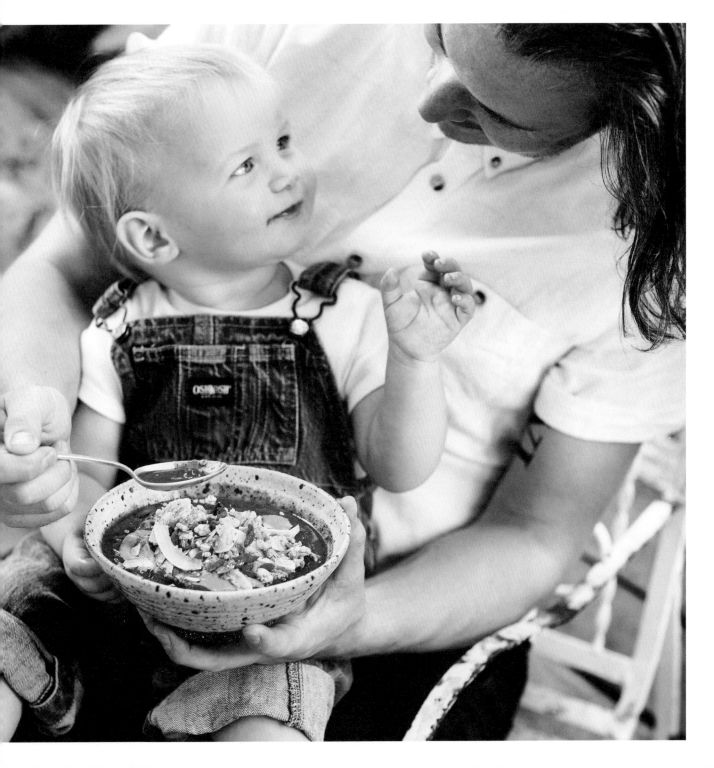

INGREDIENTS

**For the dry bircher mixture
(enough for 4–8 servings):**

300 g (10½ oz/3 cups) rolled oats

65 g (2¼ oz/½ cup) goji berries

30 g (1 oz/½ cup) finely chopped
   dried apple

2 tablespoons hemp seeds

2 tablespoons chia seeds

2 tablespoons flax seeds

2 tablespoons desiccated coconut

2 tablespoons cacao nibs

1 teaspoon powdered vanilla
   extract (optional)

For 1 portion of bircher:

60–100 g (2–3½ oz/½–1 cup)
   dry bircher mixture

120–250 ml (4–8½ fl oz/½–1 cup)
   plant milk or fruit juice

1 teaspoon maple syrup (optional)

plant-based yoghurt and fresh
fruit, to serve

Bircher

It's no secret that I'm obsessed with oats. They are high in iron and when combined with omega-rich seeds, magnesium-rich cacao nibs and antioxidant-rich goji berries, you have yourself a supremely nutritious meal. Having a jar of this ready to go makes healthy weekday breakfasts and snacks come together with very little effort.

I am a slave to a particular brand of soy milk here in Melbourne so that is what I use in my bircher, but oat milk, almond milk, rice milk, coconut milk, orange juice and apple juice all work beautifully as well.

1   Combine all the dry ingredients in a large mixing bowl. Stir to combine then spoon into the jar. The dry mixture will keep well like this for a few months.

2   Turn the jar on its side and roll it a few times to make sure the seeds are evenly distributed, as they have a tendency to sink to the bottom.

3   To make a single portion, place the dry bircher mixture in a bowl or jar with an equal amount of milk, plus the maple syrup, if using. Milks containing calcium are excellent in a vegan diet but I always use an unfortified plant milk with my oats as calcium is said to inhibit iron absorption (coffee, too).

4   Give it a good stir or shake, cover, and place in the refrigerator overnight. Stir in yoghurt and fresh fruit before serving.

TIP: If you find goji berries too bitter, replace with cranberries or any other dried fruit of your liking such as mango, apricot, etc., chopped into small pieces before being added to the mix.

INGREDIENTS

400 g (14 oz) tin chickpeas (garbanzos), drained and rinsed

90 g (3¼ oz/⅓ cup) vegan mayo

1 teaspoon wholegrain mustard

1 celery stalk, very thinly sliced

¼ red onion, very thinly sliced

small handful of parsley or coriander (cilantro) leaves, finely chopped

¼ teaspoon curry powder, or to taste (optional)

dried chilli (hot pepper) flakes, to taste

salt and freshly ground black pepper

lettuce leaf cups and toast, to serve (optional)

Curried Chickpea Mash

This is a quick and easy meal that I usually prepare and inhale in one fell swoop. I do an avocado version in my first book which I still really love but I crave this even on days where avos aren't plentiful and cheap, so the mayo is the hero here. I'm a big fan of raw red onion but you can absolutely leave it out or use less if you prefer, likewise with the curry powder.

1   Put the chickpeas in a bowl. Roughly mash about two thirds of them with a fork, then add the remaining ingredients to the bowl and stir to combine. Season to taste.

2   Serve the mash in lettuce cups or on toast, topped with a big lettuce leaf to hold everything in place. Or, serve as little sandwiches for an event or potluck.

> TIP: I prefer firmer, tinned chickpeas here. If cooking at home, be sure not to cook until they are mush.

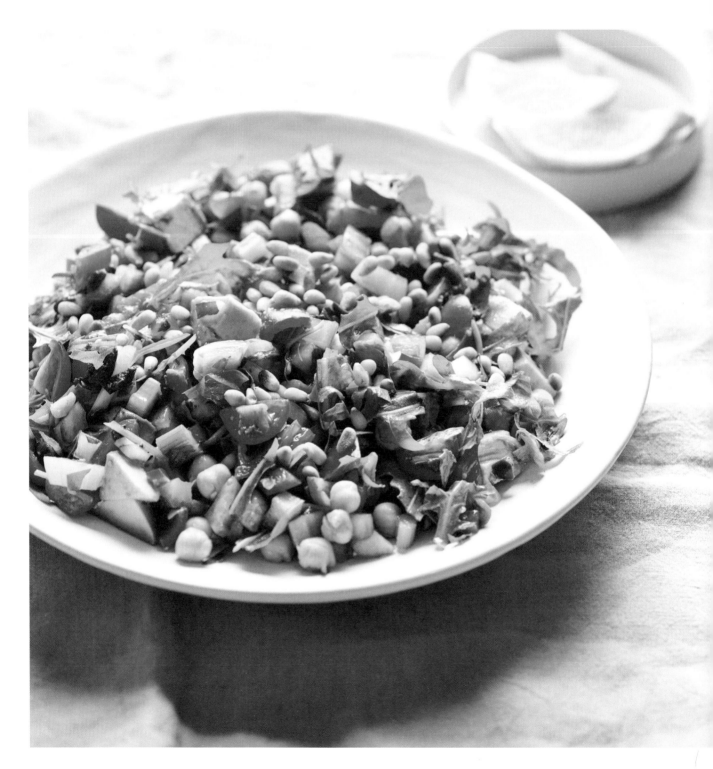

INGREDIENTS

400 g (14 oz) tin chickpeas
(garbanzos), drained
and rinsed

1 small red onion

2–3 celery stalks

1 red (bell) pepper, seeded

large handful of cherry tomatoes

small handful of pitted black olives

2 large handfuls of rocket (arugula)

1 ripe avocado

juice of 1 lemon

drizzle of olive oil

generous handful or two of my
Salad Topper (page 26) or any
other toasted seeds or nuts.
Pine nuts or almonds are my first
choice, followed by sunflower
and pumpkin seeds

Decade-old Chopped Salad

I fell in love with this salad in 2009 when I lived in New York and it's been a mainstay in my home ever since. The key to its greatness is that everything is finely chopped, so you don't end up fighting with the ingredients to get them in your mouth. If you hate chopping then this salad is not for you but I find it rather meditative and the final product never fails to hit the spot. Andy requests it for dinner often, especially on warm days.

1 Put the chickpeas in a large mixing bowl. Very finely chop the onion, celery, red pepper, tomatoes and olives, placing them in the bowl as you go.

2 Finely chop the rocket and peel, stone and dice the avocado. Add these to the bowl along with the lemon juice, olive oil and salad topper or toasted nuts or seeds. Use a spoon to give the salad a light mix, then serve.

3 Leftovers will keep in the refrigerator for up to 3–4 days.

TIP: If you want to bulk this salad up a bit to make it go further and/or increase its protein content, add up to 275 g (10 oz/scant 1½ cups) of cooked quinoa. Allow it to cool as much as possible before combining with the salad, as the heat will cause the ingredients to wilt a little and leftovers won't keep as well. If you are allergic to nuts, use seeds instead.

INGREDIENTS

150 g (5 oz/1 cup) frozen peas
2 ripe avocados, peeled and diced
1 small red onion, finely chopped
handful of fresh mint leaves,
    finely chopped
handful of fresh coriander
    (cilantro) leaves, finely chopped
grated zest of ½ and juice of
    1 unwaxed lemon
½ teaspoon salt
freshly ground black pepper,
    to taste

To serve:
toast
dried chilli (hot pepper) flakes
extra chopped mint and
    coriander (cilantro)

Pea and Avocado Smash

I love this for breakfast, but it also makes a killer guacamole and is a great one to serve with corn chips when friends come over if you need to stretch your avocados a bit. If doing this, I swap the lemon zest and juice for lime, but both ways are delish.

1   Put the peas in a large heatproof mixing bowl. Cover with boiling water and allow to defrost and warm through for 5 minutes. Drain and return to the bowl, along with the flesh of one of the avocados, and mash until smooth. Add the remaining avocado, red onion, most of the herbs, lemon zest and juice, salt and pepper and stir to combine.

2   Serve on toast, topped with chilli flakes and extra herbs. It's best eaten straight away, but will keep for a day in the refrigerator.

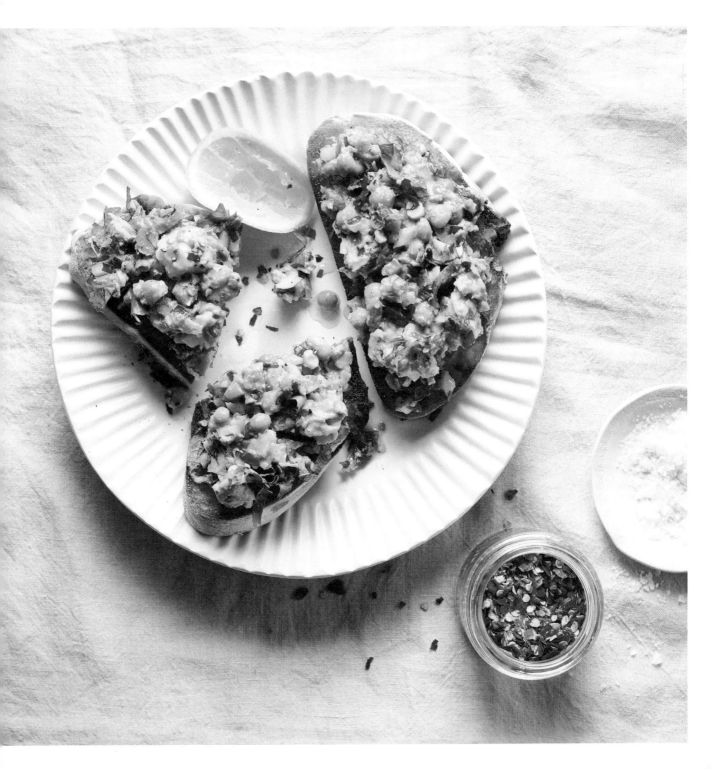

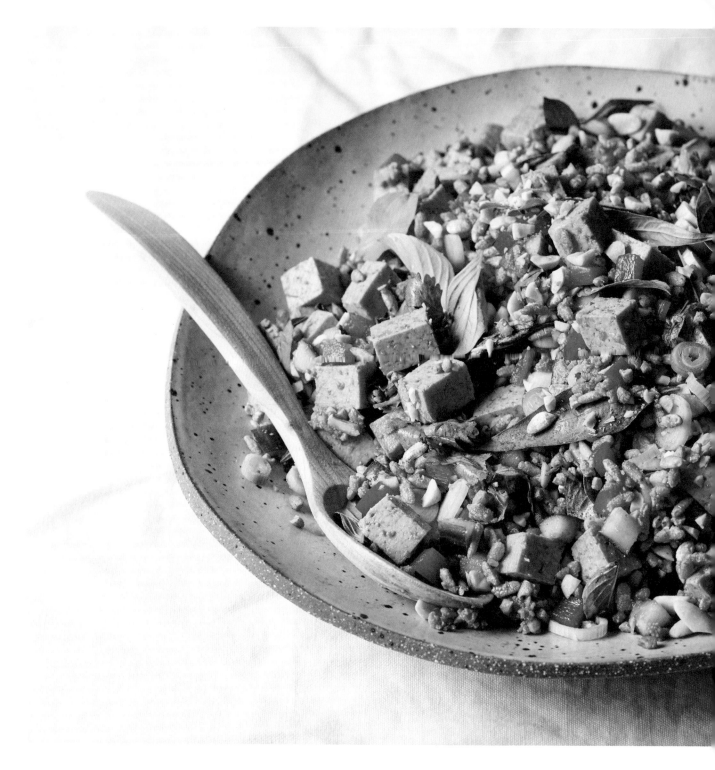

INGREDIENTS

450 g (1 lb) packet firm tofu,
  pressed and cut into 1 cm
  (½ in) pieces
3–4 spring onions (scallions),
  trimmed and finely chopped
1 cucumber, halved lengthways,
  watery core removed and
  flesh finely diced
1 red (bell) pepper, seeded
  and finely diced
80 g (3 oz/½ cup) roasted
  peanuts, roughly chopped
60 g (2 oz/1 cup firmly packed)
  leafy Asian herbs such as
  coriander (cilantro), mint,
  Thai basil, Vietnamese mint
  or basil, finely chopped
100 g (3½ oz/3½ cups) puffed
  brown rice
1 lime, halved

For the dressing:

2 tablespoons sriracha sauce
2 tablespoons tamari or soy sauce
1 tablespoon rice vinegar
1 tablespoon toasted sesame oil
1 tablespoon maple syrup
1 teaspoon tamarind paste
1 garlic clove, crushed (minced)
1 teaspoon grated fresh ginger

Spicy Peanut Puffed Rice Salad

This salad is another go-to recipe for when it's too hot to cook. I've written it as an easy recipe that doesn't require a million veggies but you can go to town on the ingredients if you are that kind of salad lover; iceberg lettuce, edamame, corn, beansprouts and avocado are all excellent additions.

You can find puffed brown rice at health food stores and some supermarkets, otherwise unsweetened breakfast rice puffs will do.

1   Combine all the dressing ingredients in a large mixing bowl and stir until well combined. Add the tofu and coat it in the dressing. Allow to sit at room temperature for at least 30 minutes, to allow time for the tofu to marinate, or all day if possible (cover the bowl with a plate and pop it in the refrigerator if that's the case).

2   When ready to serve, give the tofu a stir, then add the remaining salad ingredients (except the lime). Stir to combine, add a squeeze of fresh lime and serve immediately.

INGREDIENTS

400 g (14 oz) tin cannellini (white)
    beans, drained and rinsed
400 g (14 oz) tin chickpeas
    (garbanzos), drained
    and rinsed
400 g (14 oz) borlotti (cranberry)
    beans, drained and rinsed
½ red onion, diced
2 tomatoes, diced
1 cucumber, diced (peel if using
    a regular thick-skinned
    cucumber)
decent handful of fresh tarragon,
    leaves picked and chopped
decent handful of fresh parsley,
    leaves picked and chopped
freshly ground black pepper,
    to taste
dried chilli (hot pepper) flakes,
    to taste

For the dressing:

60 ml (2 fl oz/¼ cup) olive oil
60 ml (2 fl oz/¼ cup) red wine
    vinegar
1 small garlic clove, very finely
    chopped
1 teaspoon salt
1 teaspoon dried oregano

Tinned Bean Salad

Andy loves this salad so I try to always have a tub of it in the refrigerator that he can grab as a quick at home or work lunch. I love it too, and one of my fave dinners on a hot day is this salad paired with boiled baby potatoes doused in oil, salt, pepper, vinegar and lots of fresh tarragon.

1   Combine the dressing ingredients in a large bowl. Add the drained beans and chickpeas, veggies and herbs, and stir to combine. Add black pepper and chilli flakes to taste.

2   You can eat the salad immediately but it is much better if you let it sit in the refrigerator for a couple of hours, stirring it every now and again if you remember, so the flavours can mingle and the onion softens.

3   The salad will keep well in the refrigerator for up to 3–4 days.

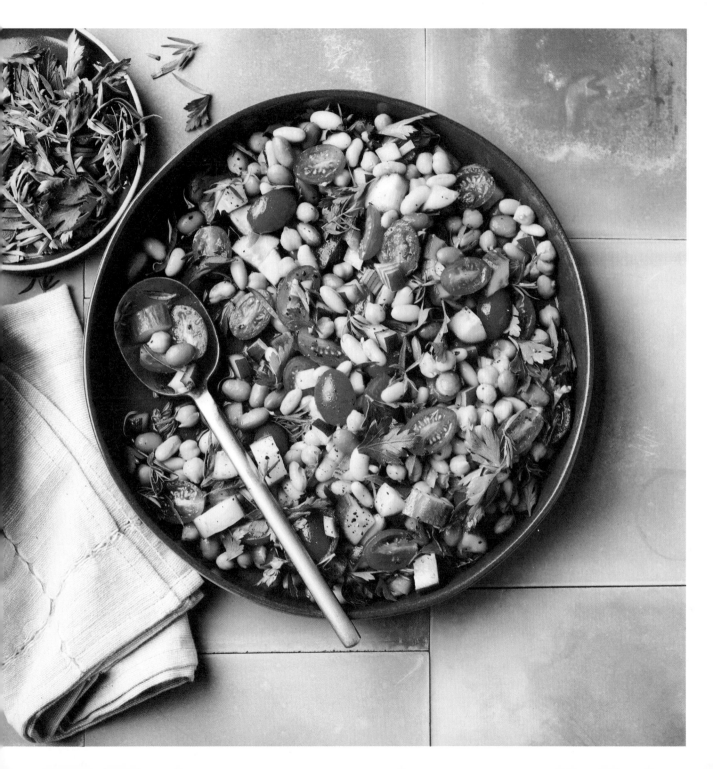

Stovetop

In this chapter you'll find things that you can prepare ahead of time and things that freeze well, make great leftovers, etc.

INGREDIENTS

For the congee:

225 g (8 oz/1 cup) short-grain
    white rice, such as koshihikari
    (or other type of sushi rice)

thumb-size piece of fresh ginger,
    peeled and thinly sliced
    (with a Microplane grater
    if you have one)

1 litre (34 fl oz/4 cups) veggie
    stock or vegan 'chicken' stock

750 ml–1 litre (25–34 fl oz/
    3–4 cups) water

½–1 teaspoon salt, to taste

For the toppings (to taste):

toasted sesame oil

tamari

toasted sesame seeds

spring onions (scallions),
    trimmed and thinly sliced

dried seaweed flakes (optional)

dried chilli (hot pepper) flakes
    (optional)

Congee

Congee is the ultimate comfort food. It's so soothing and warming, it's like getting a hug from the inside.

In this version I have kept the toppings super simple, but you can go wild with things like leftover roasted pumpkin, tofu or tempeh, sautéed greens, etc.

1   Put the rice, ginger, stock and water in a large saucepan. Bring to the boil, then reduce the heat and simmer for about 1 hour, uncovered, stirring every now and again to help the starches release from the rice. When the rice is cooked and the congee has a rice pudding like consistency add the salt, starting with half a teaspoon and adding more if you need (the final amount will depend on the saltiness of your stock).

2   Ladle the congee into bowls and top with toasted sesame oil, tamari, toasted sesame seeds, spring onions, and dried seaweed flakes and chilli, if using.

3   Leftover congee will keep well for up to a week in the refrigerator – just add a bit of water when reheating it, as congee will thicken significantly once cooled.

> TIP: I love brown rice but the point of this dish is to give your digestion a break. My friend Nina uses koshihikari rice and she makes the best congee I've ever tried, so I only use koshihikari rice in my congee too. If you can't find it easily, any short-grain rice will do, and you can absolutely use brown, or even black rice in this dish if you'd prefer.

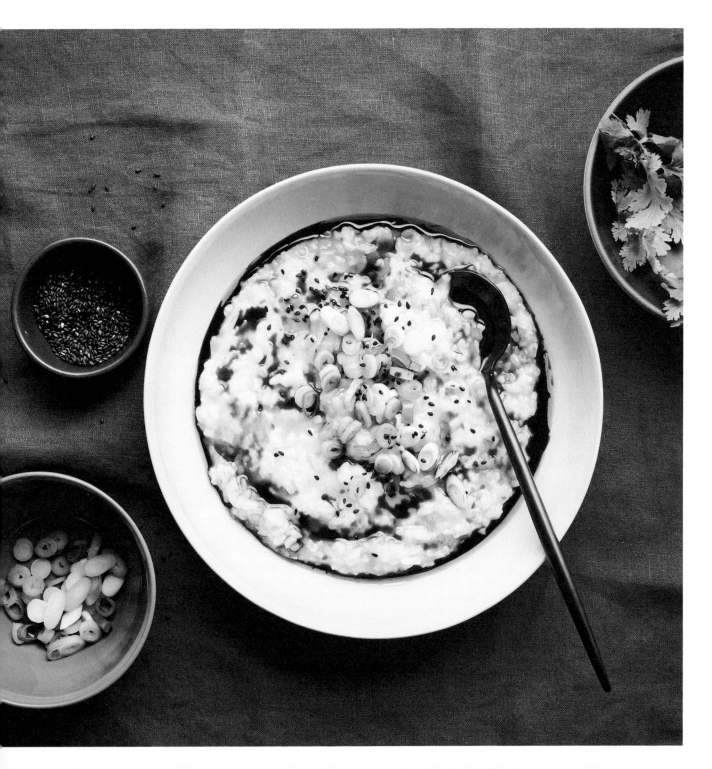

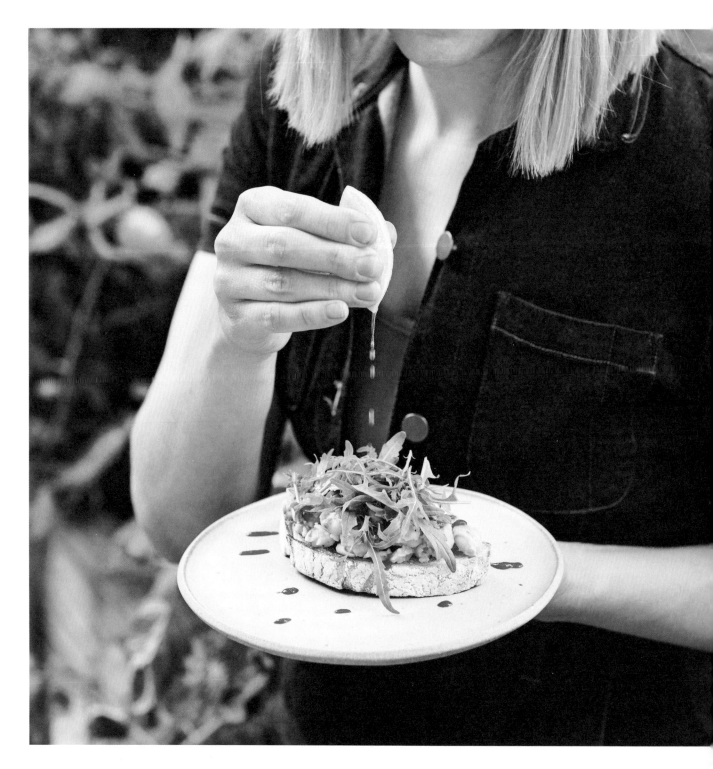

INGREDIENTS
light olive oil
1 garlic clove, finely chopped
400 g (14 oz) tin butter (lima)
    beans or cannellini (white)
    beans, drained and rinsed
squeeze of lemon juice
dried chilli (hot pepper) flakes,
    to taste
salt and freshly ground
    black pepper

Optional herbs and spices:
fresh rosemary, leaves picked
fresh thyme, leaves picked
fresh oregano, leaves picked
cumin (ground or seeds)
coriander seed
fennel seed
paprika

To serve:
toast or wrap
fresh parsley, coriander (cilantro),
    and/or fresh basil
spinach (optional)
rocket (arugula) (optional)
sundried tomatoes (optional)
tahini (optional)
grated carrot (optional)
sriracha sauce (optional)

Beans on Toast

This most basic, pantry staples version of beans on toast has been a mainstay in my home for as long as I can remember. On occasion I'll add herbs or spices but more often than not I am half dressed and one handed with a child dangling from each leg when I make this, and the most simple version is everything I need. Doused with sriracha and piled high with rocket, it never fails to hit the spot.

1   Heat a drizzle of olive oil in a frying pan (skillet) over a low heat, then add the garlic and cook for a minute or two until fragrant but not browned. If using herbs and spices, add them now, and cook for a minute or two, stirring. Then add the beans and lemon juice and mash them with a fork as they warm and soften, adding a little water to help them along and get a creamy texture.

2   Remove from the heat and serve on toast, or any other vehicle of your choosing, with a sprinkle of chilli flakes and season with salt and pepper. Keep it simple, or serve with herbs, leaves, sundried tomatoes, tahini and grated carrot.

INGREDIENTS

300 g (10½ oz/1½ cups) quinoa
750 ml (25 fl oz/3 cups) water
1 head of broccoli, cut into
    bite-size florets and stalk
    trimmed and thinly sliced
300 g (10½ oz) smoked tofu,
    cut into 1 cm (½ in) cubes
a few handfuls of rocket (arugula)
    or baby spinach, roughly
    chopped
large handful of fresh coriander
    (cilantro) or any other Asian
    herbs (such as Thai basil or
    Vietnamese mint), roughly
    chopped
2 tablespoons toasted white
    sesame seeds
dried chilli (hot pepper) flakes,
    to taste

For the dressing:

65 g (2¼ oz/¼ cup) tahini
1 heaped tablespoon white
    miso paste
2 tablespoons rice vinegar
1 tablespoon tamari
1 teaspoon finely grated fresh
    ginger (with a Microplane grater
    if you have one)
120 ml (4 fl oz/½ cup) warm water

Miso Tahini Quinoa

When I asked Andy what his favourite meal of 2019 was, he said this. We ate it a lot, and in many variations, but both agree that the smoked tofu and broccoli version is the one that is worthy of cookbook real estate. If you can't find smoked tofu I recommend subbing with frozen and shelled edamame as opposed to plain, unmarinated, unsmoked tofu which is flavourless and doesn't work in this dish at all.

1 Rinse the quinoa in a sieve (fine mesh strainer) under cold running water then put it in a large saucepan with the water. Cover with a lid and bring to the boil then reduce the heat and simmer for 15 minutes.

2 After 15 minutes, add the broccoli (florets and sliced stalk) and tofu to the pan and cover again with the lid. Allow to cook for a further 5 minutes, until all the water has been absorbed. Resist the urge to stir it at this point, as quinoa is best left undisturbed until it has finished cooking.

3 To make the dressing, put all the ingredients into a screw-top lidded jar, screw the lid on and shake well until combined.

4 Remove the pan from the heat, stir and allow to sit, covered, for another 5 minutes, then drizzle with three-quarters of the dressing. Stir to combine. Add the rocket or spinach and coriander and serve (warm or cool), topped with toasted sesame seeds, chilli flakes and the remaining dressing.

5 Leftovers will keep well in the refrigerator for up to 3 days.

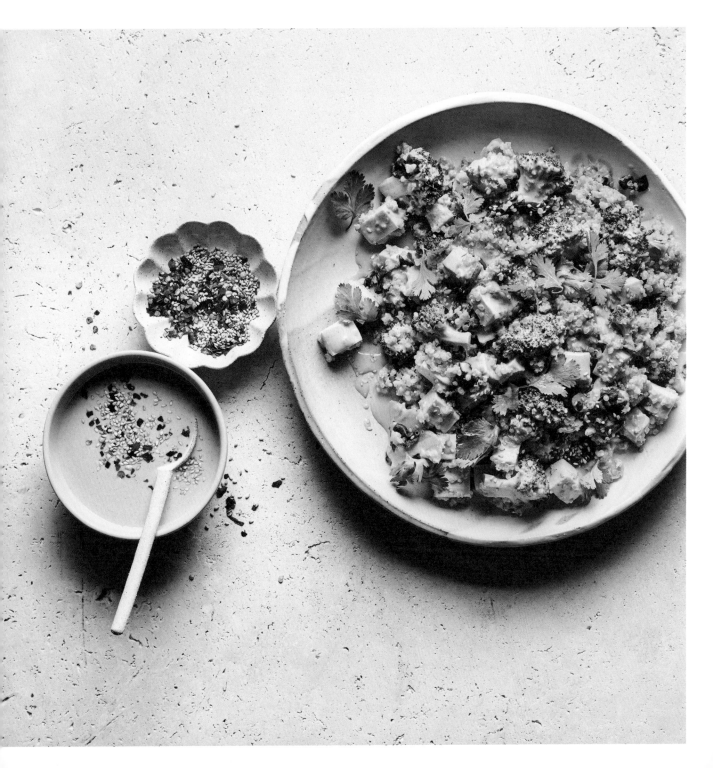

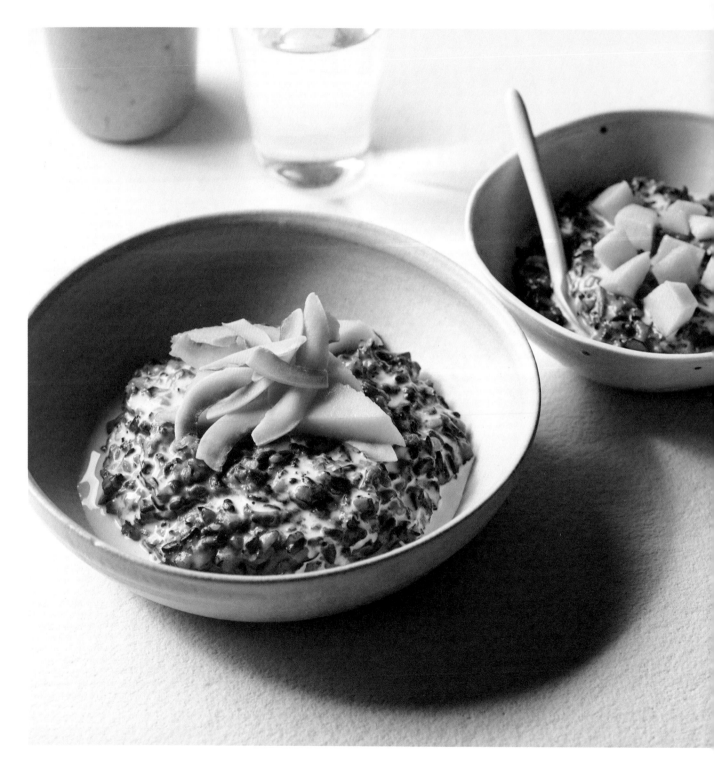

SERVES 2–4

INGREDIENTS
185 g (6½ oz/1 cup) black rice
750 ml (25 fl oz/3 cups) water
pinch of salt
400 ml (14 fl oz) tin coconut milk
4 Medjool dates, or 8 Deglet Noor
   dates, stoned and finely
   chopped
1 tablespoon vanilla extract

To serve:
sliced banana, mango
   or other fresh fruit
toasted flaked (sliced)
   coconut (optional)

Date and Coconut Black Rice Pudding

When I was heavily pregnant with Louie I was making black rice pudding a LOT. The black rice I used in Berlin was super black and one day when getting ready to run some errands, I snarfed a few mouthfuls of this on my way out the door. A few hours later, after speaking bad German to anyone who would look at me, I came home to see my teeth and corners of my mouth FILLED with black rice. To this day I still think about this incident and laugh to myself whenever I eat black rice pudding.

1 Soak the rice in a medium saucepan of cold water overnight.

2 The next day, drain the rice, return it to the pan, add the water and salt, cover and bring to the boil, then reduce the heat to low and simmer for 45 minutes. The water should be almost, but not quite absorbed.

3 Add 300 ml (10 fl oz/1¼ cups) of the coconut milk, along with the chopped dates and vanilla, stir to combine, then replace the lid and cook for a further 20 minutes. Remove from heat, uncover and allow to sit for 10 minutes then stir once more and spoon into bowls.

4 Top with the remaining coconut milk, some fresh fruit and toasted coconut flakes (if using). Enjoy immediately and store any leftovers in the refrigerator – they will keep well for a few days.

INGREDIENTS
250 g (9 oz) podded fresh
    of frozen broad (fava) beans
glug of olive oil
½ lemon
60 g (2 oz) good-quality
    vegan feta
small handful of fresh parsley
    leaves, finely chopped
salt and freshly ground
    black pepper
dried chilli (hot pepper) flakes
toast, to serve (optional)

The Simplest Broad Beans

If you know me then you know about my neighbour from three doors down, who leaves giant bags of veggies on my doorstep all year round. Her broad beans were the first I ever cooked from scratch and I'm so glad I did so before writing this book. What a treat! They are the most perfect beings in all of their tender simplicity, and I'm hooked! If, like me, you have been intimidated by broad beans all your life, wait no more. Find some, shell them, boil them and shell them again before serving with the best quality olive oil and feta you can find. It's beyond worth it.

1   Blanch the beans in a saucepan of boiling water for 3 minutes. Drain and allow to cool, or immerse in a bowl of ice-cold water to speed up the cooling process. Remove the outer lighter-coloured pod to reveal the vibrant green pod on the inside.

2   Once you have podded all of your beans, simply toss them in a bowl with the oil, a squeeze of lemon juice, crumble over the vegan feta, sprinkle over the parsley and season with a pinch each of salt and pepper, and chilli flakes to taste. Serve on toast or eat straight from the bowl. So simple, so delish.

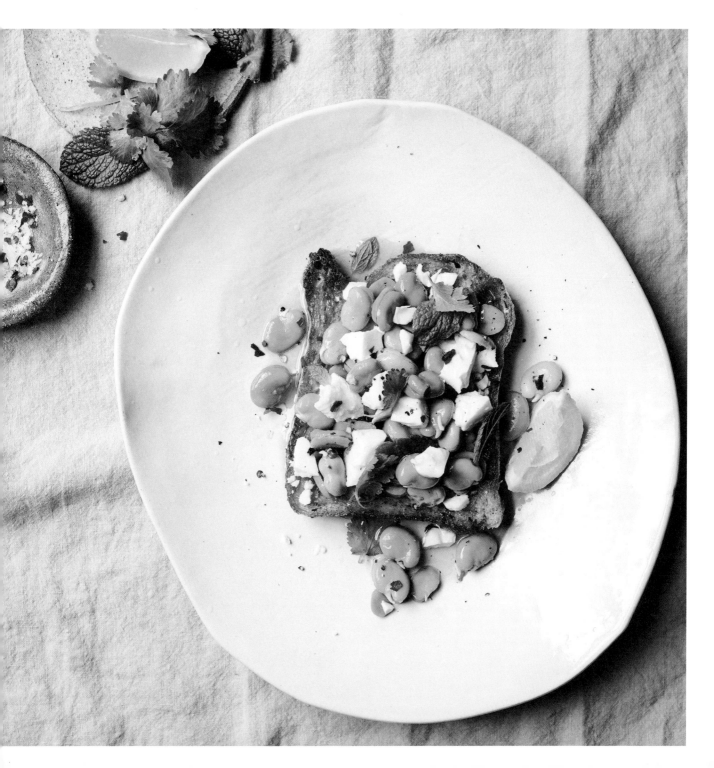

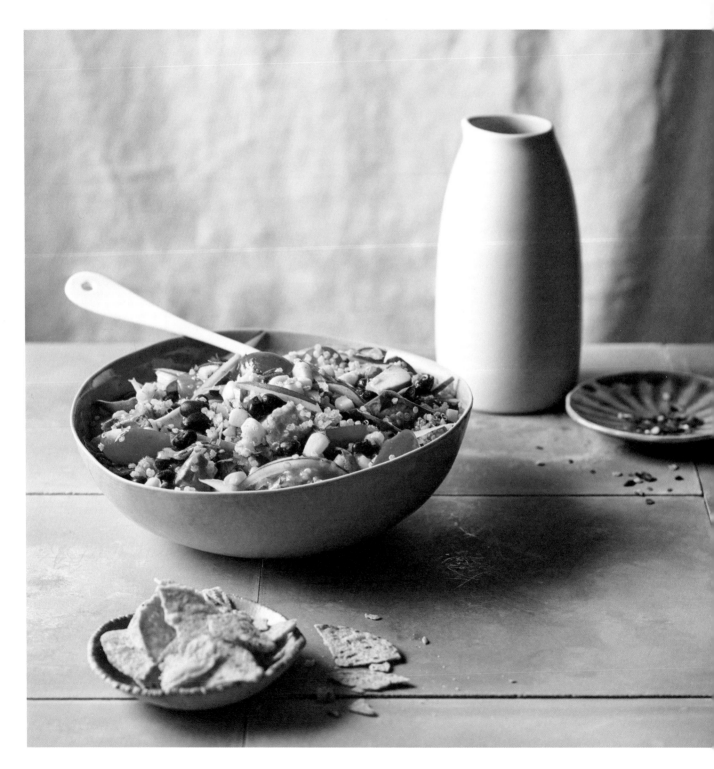

INGREDIENTS
200 g (7 oz/1 cup) quinoa
500 ml (17 fl oz/2 cups) water
½ teaspoon salt, plus extra
    to season the finished salad
olive oil, for drizzling
1 teaspoon sweet smoked paprika
1 teaspoon cumin seeds
1 ripe avocado, peeled and diced
400 g (14 oz) tin black beans,
    drained and rinsed
400 g (14 oz) tin sweetcorn,
    drained and rinsed
1 red onion, thinly sliced
200 g (7 oz) cherry tomatoes,
    halved or quartered
3–4 handfuls of leafy greens –
    I like to use a combination
    of rocket (arugula) and spinach –
    larger leaves chopped
handful of fresh coriander (cilantro)
    leaves, finely chopped

For the dressing:
60 ml (2 fl oz/¼ cup) olive oil
2 tablespoons tamarind paste (see Tip)
2 tablespoons water
1 tablespoon maple syrup
1 garlic clove, crushed (minced)
½ teaspoon salt

To serve (optional):
a few handfuls of plain salted,
    organic corn chips, crushed
a few tablespoons of something
    creamy such as vegan sour cream
    or Cashew Cream (page 22), thinned
    to a pourable consistency

Mexi Quinoa Salad

This salad is the bomb. It's easy, yum, and keeps for days, even with corn chips crunched into it which are surprisingly moreish when they go a bit soggy. Combine it with Black Bean Soup (page 86) for a hearty combo to serve a crowd or sustain you for a good number of days.

1 Rinse the quinoa in a sieve (fine mesh strainer) under cold running water then put it in a small saucepan with the water and the salt. Cover, bring to the boil, then reduce the heat and simmer for 20 minutes, until all the water has been absorbed. Remove from the heat, take off the lid, and add a light drizzle of olive oil, the smoked paprika and cumin seeds. Fluff the grains with a fork and allow to sit, uncovered, for 10 minutes.

2 While the quinoa is cooking and cooling, prepare the dressing by combining all the ingredients in a small bowl or lidded screw-top glass jar and whisking or shaking to combine.

3 Once the quinoa has cooled, add the remaining salad ingredients and stir to combine. Add the dressing and stir once more, then spoon into bowls and top with crushed corn chips and drizzle with something creamy (if using).

4 Eat straight away, or store in an airtight container. It will keep well in the refrigerator for a couple of days, even if you added corn chips, which are actually really incredibly delicious when they get a bit soggy.

> TIP: If you don't have tamarind paste, use the juice of 2 limes in place of the tamarind and water.

INGREDIENTS

2 tablespoons coconut oil

400–500 g (14 oz–1 lb 2 oz) firm tofu
(doesn't need to be pressed)

4 tablespoons Scrambled Tofu
Seasoning (page 27)

KALA NAMAK/
BLACK SALT

This salt is the absolute
bomb. Hailed by Ayurvedic
practitioners for its
medicinal qualities, it
contains sulphur, which
lends an eggy flavour
to your tofu scramble.
Depending on where you
live, it may be hard to find,
but I am noticing it pop up
in more and more health
food and Asian stores, so
even if you haven't heard
of it before, you may be
surprised how easy it is to
source. If you can't find it,
standard salt will do and
your scramble will still
be delicious.

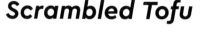

Scrambled Tofu

Scrambled tofu is delicious, filling, infinitely customisable and when you have the spice mix made already it comes together in moments. I cook it often, as others would eggs, for a quick and easy meal at any time of day.

In many of my recipes I call for pressing tofu before cooking with it; however, this one is an exception as the liquid in the tofu helps to prevent the tofu sticking to the pan.

1   Heat the coconut oil in frying pan (skillet) over a medium-high heat. Crumble in the tofu and toss over the heat for about 5 minutes. When the tofu starts to brown, add the tofu seasoning and use a spatula to stir and toss it until the tofu is coated in the spices – gently, as you want the occasional chunk to remain. Continue cooking for about 5 minutes until light golden brown, then add any extra ingredients, if using.

2   Remove from the heat and serve the scrambled tofu as it is, or use any of the serving ideas listed below.

SERVING IDEAS

- On toast with avocado or hummus and rocket (arugula).
- In a Breakfast Burrito (page 61).
- In tacos with black beans, Really Good Potatoes (page 135) and spinach.
- In a bowl with cooked quinoa and rocket.
- On a bagel with avocado and coconut 'bacon'.

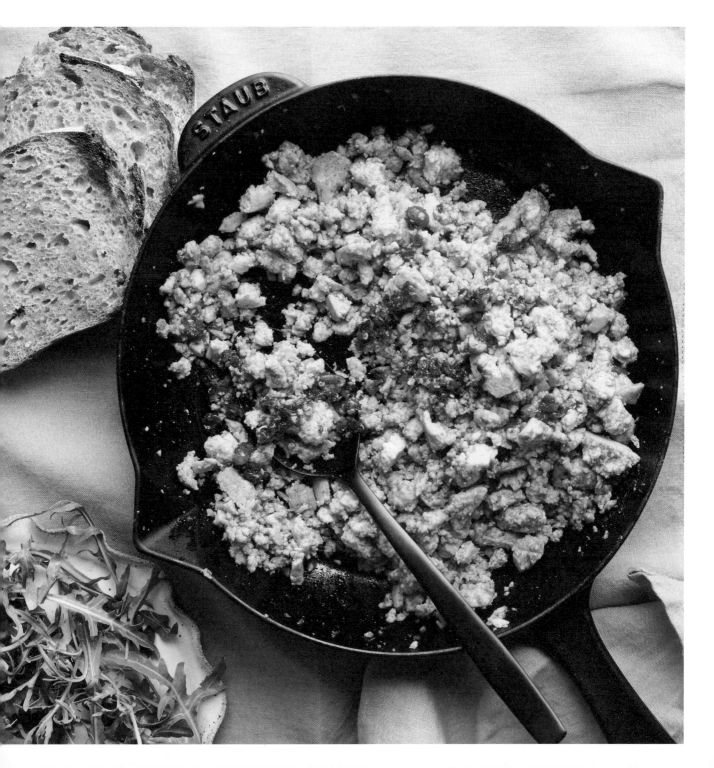

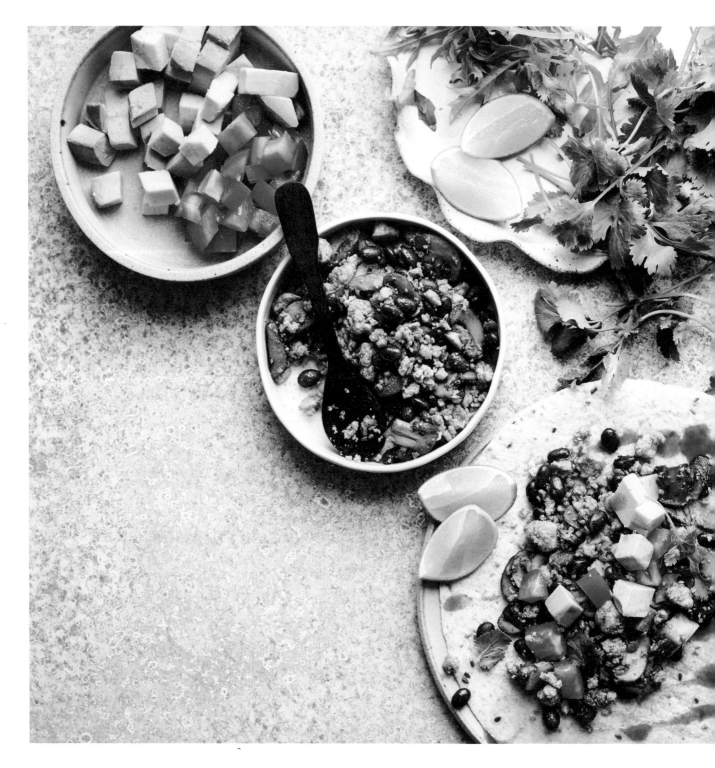

INGREDIENTS

olive oil, for frying

300 g (10½ oz) mushrooms,
  cleaned and very thinly sliced

375 g (13 oz) firm tofu, drained and
  crumbled (no need to press)

4 tablespoons Scrambled Tofu
  Seasoning (page 27)

400 g (14 oz) tin black beans,
  drained and rinsed (or 260 g/
  9½ oz/1½ cups Beloved Black
  Beans – page 74)

4 large wheat wraps

4–8 tablespoons Cashew
  Cream (page 22) or good-
  quality vegan cream cheese,
  sour cream or even straight-up
  vegan cheese

a few handfuls of rocket (arugula)
  or other leafy salad green

1 large tomato, diced

1 ripe avocado, peeled and
  diced (optional)

handful of fresh coriander
  (cilantro), roughly chopped
  (optional)

hot sauce, to taste

salt

Mushroom and Black Bean Breakfast Burritos

Breakfast burritos are a staple in our home, and not just for breakfast. We make a few different versions, and enjoy them for dinner just as often as we do for breakfast and lunch, but Andy and I both agree that this Mushroom and Black Bean version is the best of the best.

1   Heat a large frying pan (skillet) over a medium-high heat. Add enough oil to coat the bottom, then add the mushrooms and a pinch of salt and cook for a good 10 minutes, until the liquid from the mushrooms has been released and evaporated.

2   Push the mushrooms to the side of the pan, add more oil to coat the bottom of the pan, then add the crumbled tofu and cook for 5–10 minutes, stirring frequently, until the tofu starts to brown – it's okay to start to incorporate the mushrooms into the tofu at this point. Once the tofu has started to brown, add the tofu seasoning and stir to coat the tofu mixture evenly, then add the black beans and cook for another 5 minutes or so, until the beans are warm. If the mixture starts to stick to the base of the pan at any stage, add a little water.

3   Once your filling is ready, heat your wraps in the microwave on one of the plates you'll be eating from.

4   Smear each warmed wrap with Cashew Cream. Add the rocket, warm bean and mushroom filling, diced tomato, diced avocado and coriander, if using, and hot sauce. Fold into a burrito and enjoy immediately. Any leftover bean mix will store well in the refrigerator in an airtight container for a couple of days.

TIP: If you don't have access to black salt to make the Scrambled Tofu Seasoning, use the Really Good Potato seasoning instead (page 27).

INGREDIENTS

For the sauce:
1 tablespoon toasted sesame oil
1 tablespoon rice vinegar
1 tablespoon sambal oelek
1 teaspoon maple syrup
4 tablespoons tamari

For the filling:
3 tablespoons peanut or coconut oil
3 spring onions (scallions), trimmed
    and white parts cut into thin rounds
thumb-size piece of fresh ginger,
    peeled and finely chopped
2 garlic cloves, finely chopped
150 g (5 oz) assorted mushrooms,
    cleaned and finely chopped
    (no need to be too exact in the
    chopping)
450 g (1 lb) firm tofu, drained
    and pressed, then crumbled
1 tablespoon toasted black
    sesame seeds

To serve:
2 heads gem (bibb) or baby cos
    lettuce leaves, separated,
    washed and dried
handful each of fresh Asian herbs such
    as Thai basil, Vietnamese mint and
    coriander (cilantro), leaves picked

Mushroom and Tofu San Choy Bau

San Choy Bau is the perfect summer food and I crave it when I want something warm and filling but refreshing and light. If you haven't cooked with Thai basil or Vietnamese mint, I implore you to try them as their flavours are really what makes this dish.

1   Mix all the sauce ingredients together in a small cup or jar and set aside.

2   Heat the peanut or coconut oil in a large frying pan (skillet) over a medium-high heat. Add the spring onions and ginger and cook for a couple of minutes until fragrant, then add the garlic, mushrooms and tofu and cook for 5–10 minutes, stirring frequently, until all of the liquid from the mushrooms has been released and has evaporated.

3   Stir in the sauce and cook for a further 5 minutes until the tofu starts to brown. Then, stir in the sesame seeds, remove from the heat and spoon the filling into lettuce cups. Garnish with fresh herbs to serve. Any leftover tofu mixture will keep well in the refrigerator for up to 2 days.

> TIP: This also goes amazingly with noodles. I like to cut my mushrooms into thin slices when serving this way, and with wide rice noodles that cook by soaking in water that I can then just chuck in the pan along with the herbs, and toss to combine.

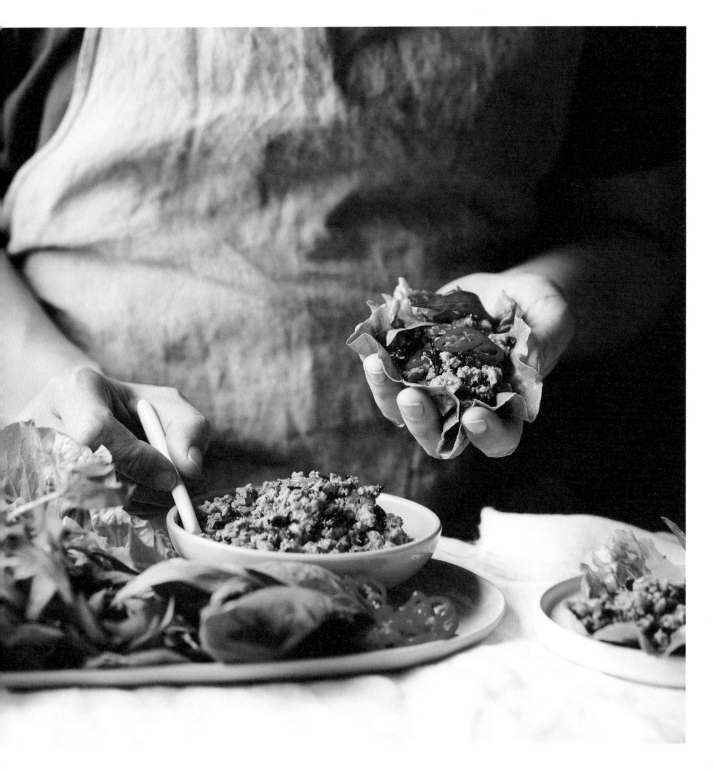

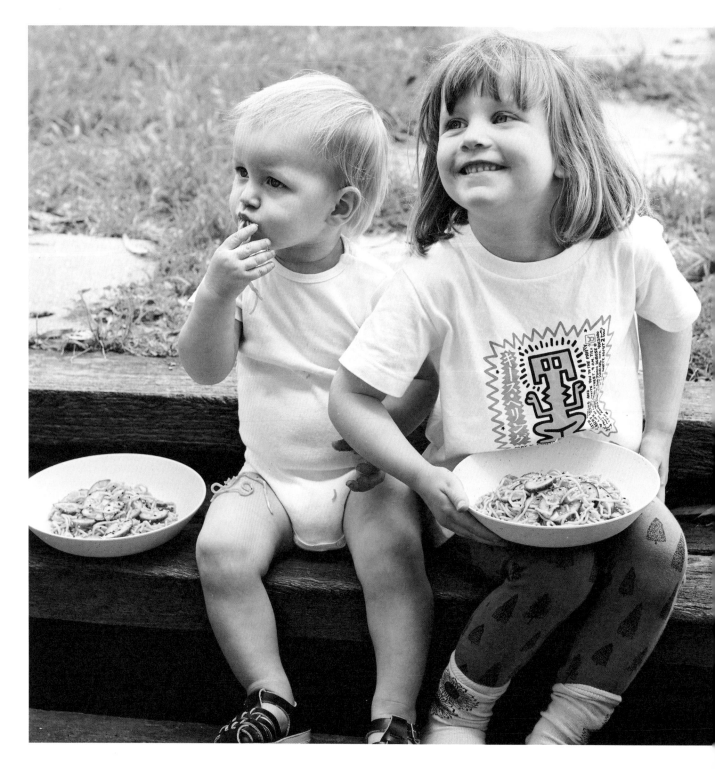

INGREDIENTS

about 250 g (9 oz) dried noodles

2 tablespoons tamari

1 tablespoon rice vinegar

1 tablespoon toasted sesame oil

1 tablespoon maple syrup

2 tablespoons toasted sesame seeds

3–4 spring onions (scallions), trimmed and thinly sliced (optional)

1 teaspoon finely grated fresh ginger (optional)

1 teaspoon finely grated garlic (optional)

1 cucumber, halved lengthways and thinly sliced on the diagonal (peel the cucumber if it has thick skin)

chilli oil or sriracha sauce, to taste

Quickest Noodles

You know when its hot and you wanna eat something but want it to be fast and simple and maybe not even have any veggies? This is what you need to make. The sauce goes with any noodles, and I always have a packet or five floating around my pantry. If I am in the mood I'll add some tofu or edamame, but this dish is mostly reserved for evenings when I've had a lot to eat that day and just want a light and gentle dinner.

1   Bring a medium saucepan of water to the boil over a high heat. Add the noodles and cook according to the packet instructions.

2   While the noodles are cooking, combine the tamari, rice vinegar, sesame oil and maple syrup in a small cup or jar and stir to combine.

3   Drain the cooked noodles and put them back in the pan along with the sauce, toasted sesame seeds, spring onions, ginger and garlic (if using). Toss so that the noodles are well coated, then add the cucumber and toss once more. Spoon into bowls and top with chilli oil or sriracha.

INGREDIENTS
2 tablespoons olive oil
2–3 garlic cloves, finely chopped
1 teaspoon flaky salt
450 g (1 lb) mushrooms, cleaned
    and cut into 2.5 cm (1 in) dice
3–4 sprigs of fresh lemon thyme
pinch of ground or freshly grated
    nutmeg (optional but so good)
generous tablespoon of pesto
    (try my Green Pesto on page 21)
    or good-quality soft (vegan)
    cheese
fresh or toasted bread, to serve

Mum's Mushrooms

Every time my mum comes to stay with me, she makes a big pan of mushrooms and eats them with toasted sourdough that I have lovingly prepared for her arrival. She especially loves king oyster mushrooms, which are difficult to find where she lives. I grow lemon thyme in my garden to serve with mushrooms, because there is no better combo in my opinion. We like to cook them low and slow, and then add something creamy at the end – either a dollop of soft (vegan) cheese or a spoonful of pesto, or both.

1   Heat the oil in a large frying pan (skillet) over a medium heat. Add the garlic and salt and cook for a couple of minutes until the garlic is fragrant but not browned, then add the mushrooms, lemon thyme and nutmeg, and cook for at least 10 minutes, stirring every so often but mainly leaving them to their own devices. First they will release their liquid, then they will slowly caramelise in the pan. Of course, you can cook them more quickly if you are in a hurry, but the lower and slower the better, in my opinion.

2   Once cooked, remove from the heat and stir through the pesto or soft cheese if using, and toast your bread (if toasting).

3   Serve the mushrooms in bowls or on a plate, with bread.

TIP: As well as being a favourite comfort food meal, these mushrooms make a killer addition to most of the recipes in this chapter. Andy eats them in a wrap, with lettuce. They are incredible with hummus or white bean mash, Scrambled Tofu (page 58), to accompany fritters, etc.

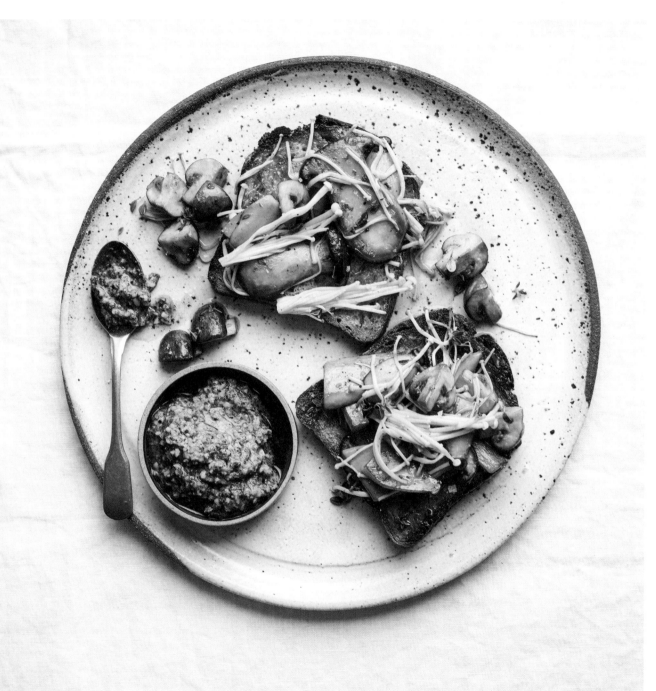

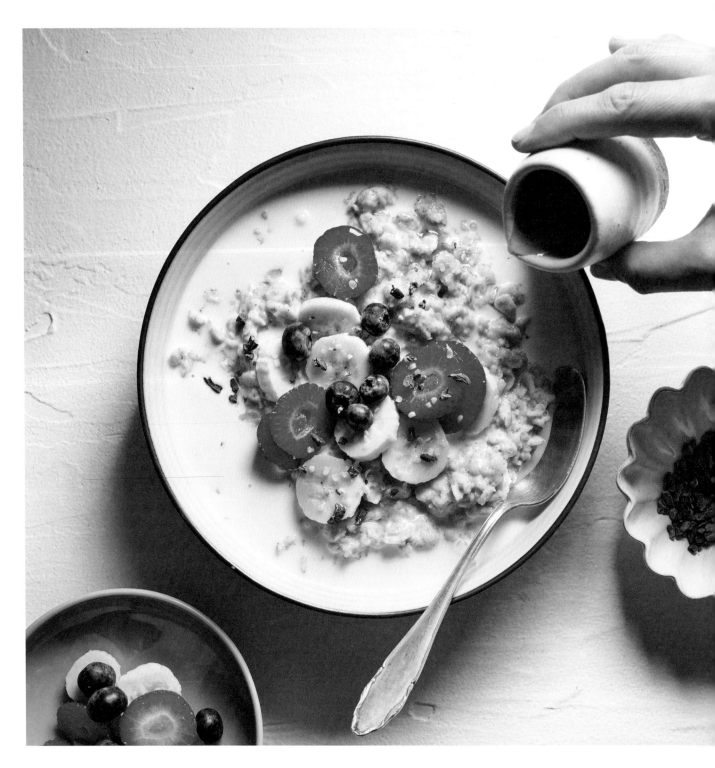

INGREDIENTS
100 g (3½ oz/1 cup) rolled oats
or quick-cook oats
250 ml (8½ fl oz/1 cup) water
250 ml (8½ fl oz/1 cup) soy,
coconut or almond milk,
plus extra for topping
1 tablespoon LSA (mixture
of linseed, sunflower seeds
and almonds)
½ teaspoon ground cinnamon
(optional)
½ teaspoon vanilla extract
(optional)
¼ teaspoon ground nutmeg
(optional)

For the toppings:
seasonal fruit, cacao nibs,
nut butters, syrup, nuts,
seeds, etc.

Just Your Everyday Porridge

A full blown porridge mania has swept the food world over the past few years. As well as boasting an impressive nutritional profile, oats are easy to cook and when turned into porridge, this humble superfood provides a perfect canvas for the most simple or decadent of toppings.

There are a million and one porridge recipes out there, but this one is my go-to. I love it, my kids love it, and the addition of healthy fats means it keeps me full for hours.

1 Put the oats, water, milk, LSA and spices (if using) in a small saucepan. Bring to the boil then reduce the heat to a gentle simmer and cook, stirring frequently, until the liquid is absorbed and you have a smooth and creamy porridge.

2 Spoon into a bowl (or bowls) and top with extra milk and whichever toppings your heart desires. In the picture I've used banana, strawberry, blueberry, hemp seeds and cacao nibs, with a generous drizzle of maple syrup.

TIP: Oats contain iron which is best absorbed if you eat it with vitamin C, so adding blueberries or some other kind of vitamin C rich fruit is a great idea. If possible, avoid calcium fortified milks for your porridge as calcium inhibits the absorption of iron.

INGREDIENTS
270 g (10 oz) soba (buckwheat)
 or udon noodles
200 g (7 oz) shelled frozen
 edamame, thawed
200 g (7 oz) baby spinach
1 ripe avocado, peeled and diced
3 tablespoons toasted sesame
 seeds
2 tablespoons finely chopped
 fresh coriander (cilantro), plus
 extra to garnish (optional)
5 fresh kaffir lime leaves,
 thinly sliced
fresh chilli, thinly sliced, to garnish

For the satay sauce:
125 g (4 oz/½ cup) smooth
 peanut butter
60 ml (2 fl oz/¼ cup) tamari
2 tablespoons maple syrup
1 teaspoon tamarind paste
100 ml (3½ fl oz/scant ½ cup)
 warm water

Satay Noodles

This is a household favourite that comes together in minutes once you've got your water boiling. If you aren't familiar with kaffir lime leaves, don't be put off by their inclusion in this recipe! They are easier to find than you think and once you've tried them you'll want to use them in everything. There are very rarely any leftovers for this dish, but if there are they are delicious both hot and cold.

Of course, substitute the udon or soba noodles for any noodles you like; however, thick are better, as they hold the heavy ingredients more easily.

1   Bring a large saucepan of water to the boil.

2   While you are waiting for the water to boil, make the satay sauce by combining the peanut butter, tamari, maple syrup and tamarind paste in a small bowl. Add the warm water and stir. It should be thick but slightly runny. If it seems too thick, add more warm water, 1 tablespoon at a time, until the desired consistency is reached (the amount of water you need will depend on the consistency of your peanut butter). Set aside.

3   Once the water is boiling, add the noodles and cook according to the packet instructions. Add the thawed edamame for the final minute and the spinach for the final 30 seconds. Drain in a colander and shake to remove excess water. Return the noodles, edamame and spinach to the pan and add the dressing, diced avocado, sesame seeds, coriander and kaffir lime leaves. Toss to combine then serve in bowls, garnished with fresh chilli and additional coriander, if you're a fan.

TIP: You can make the sauce ahead of time and it will keep for a few days in an airtight container in the fridge.

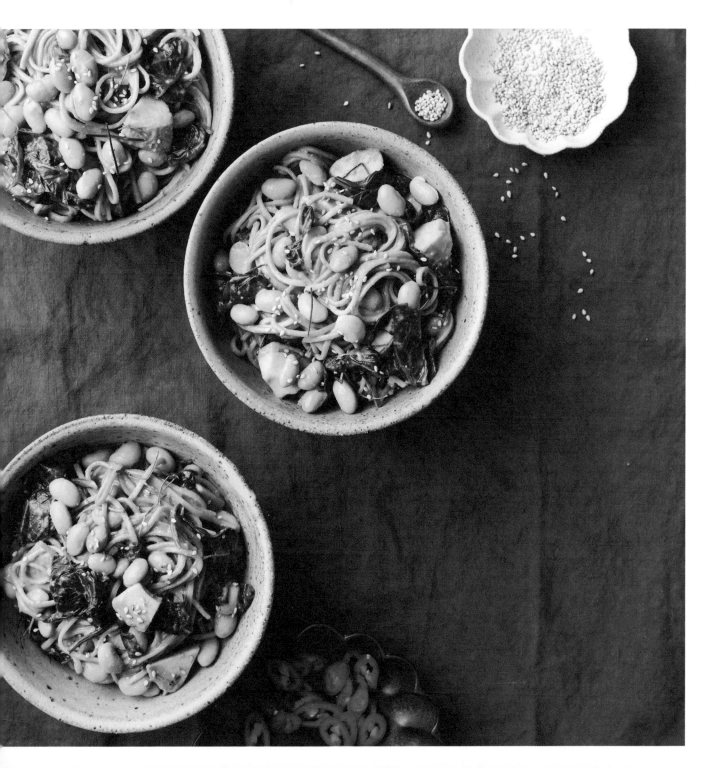

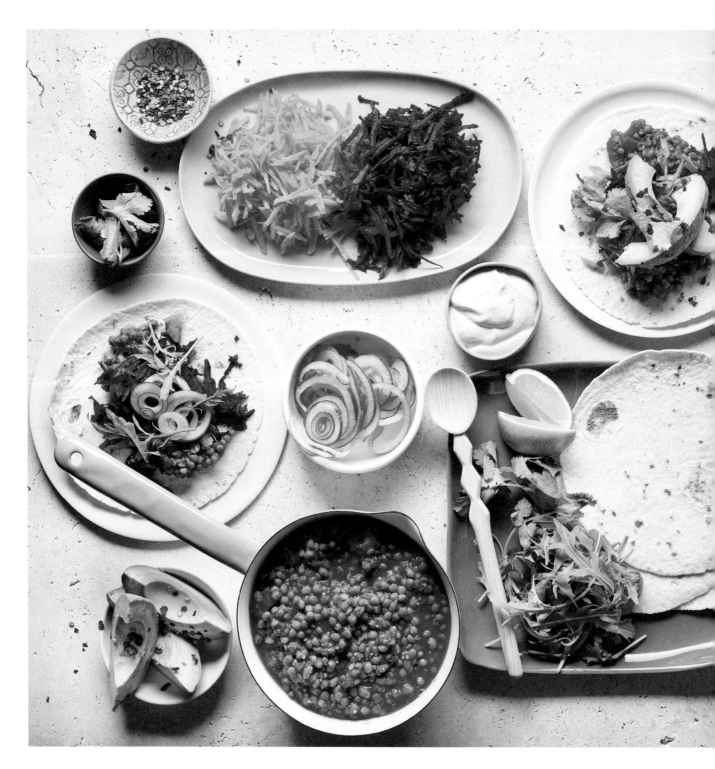

INGREDIENTS

For the lentils:

2 × 400 g (14 oz) tins of lentils (green or brown), drained and rinsed

400 g (14 oz) tin chopped tomatoes

1 chipotle pepper in adobo, chopped, plus 1 tablespoon of the sauce

1 teaspoon onion powder

1 teaspoon garlic powder

1 teaspoon salt

large handful of fresh coriander (cilantro) leaves, finely chopped

For the tacos:

12 soft-shell wheat or corn tacos

a few handfuls of fresh leaves and vegetables such as rocket (arugula), grated carrot, grated beetroot (beets), etc.

1 ripe avocado, peeled and cut into wedges

3–4 tablespoons something creamy such as Cashew Cream (page 22) or good-quality vegan sour cream

1–2 limes, halved, for juicing

The Quickest and Easiest Smoky Lentil Tacos

Black beans are and forever will be my favourite taco filling, however tinned lentils have a very special place in my heart too, due to their sheer ease and ability to come together in moments.

For the toppings, you can use whatever you like, but to keep the chopping to an absolute minimum I usually use something leafy like rocket or baby spinach, and something I can quickly grate such as carrot or beetroot (beets).

The lentils can be eaten immediately or left for a few days and reheated as needed. They can also be spooned onto baked sweet potatoes, over rice, in burritos, etc.

1   First, prepare the lentils. Put the lentils in a medium-large saucepan with the chopped tomatoes, chipotle, onion powder, garlic powder and salt. Stir to combine and allow to heat through for a few minutes while you gather and prepare the rest of your ingredients. Once warm, stir in the coriander.

2   Spoon the lentils onto tacos and top with some leaves and vegetables of your choice plus some avocado and whichever fresh and creamy ingredients you are using, and squeeze over some lime juice. Devour.

TIP: Do try to get your hands on chipotles in adobo. They last forever and have the ability to take a meal from mediocre to incredible.

INGREDIENTS

440 g (15½ oz/2 cups) dried black beans, rinsed and checked for stones

2 litres (70 fl oz/8 cups) water

1 onion, diced

2–3 garlic cloves, crushed (minced)

2 teaspoons salt

2 teaspoons ground cumin

2 teaspoons ground coriander

2 chipotle peppers in adobo, chopped (optional)

Beloved Black Beans

If I could eat only one thing for the rest of my life, black beans would be it. By far the most delicious of all the beans, I first discovered them when I was living in New York in 2009, and when I returned 'home' to Australia, they were really tricky to find. In the decade since then, they have grown in popularity to the point where you can even find them in tins at big chain supermarkets. Praise be!

I don't soak my dried beans before cooking them which is a nutritional no-no (soaking pulses breaks down their phytic acid which is an important step if you want to maximise nutrient absorption), but I skip this step for two reasons – the first being that black beans cook really quickly without presoaking and the second being that soaking them washes away the black sediment that gives them such an incredible flavour.

You can throw a pot of these beans on at any time of the day; in the morning to enjoy as a warm lunch and then dinner that night, or even while cooking dinner, to then enjoy the following day. They freeze beautifully too.

I usually eat a bowl of these as soon as they are cooked, topped with cashew cream, coriander and nothing else. They then get turned into an array of other meals which will do fine with tinned beans but will be orgasmic if you use these ones. Think nachos, burritos, beans and rice, tacos, anything except salad, where firmer, whole beans would be preferable.

1   Put the beans and water in a large saucepan and bring to the boil. Once boiling, add the onion, garlic, salt, spices and peppers (if using). Reduce the heat and simmer uncovered for 1½–2 hours, until beans are very easy to squish on the side of the pan with the back of a spoon. You can serve them as is, or use a potato masher to mash them gently so that they thicken a little.

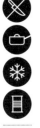

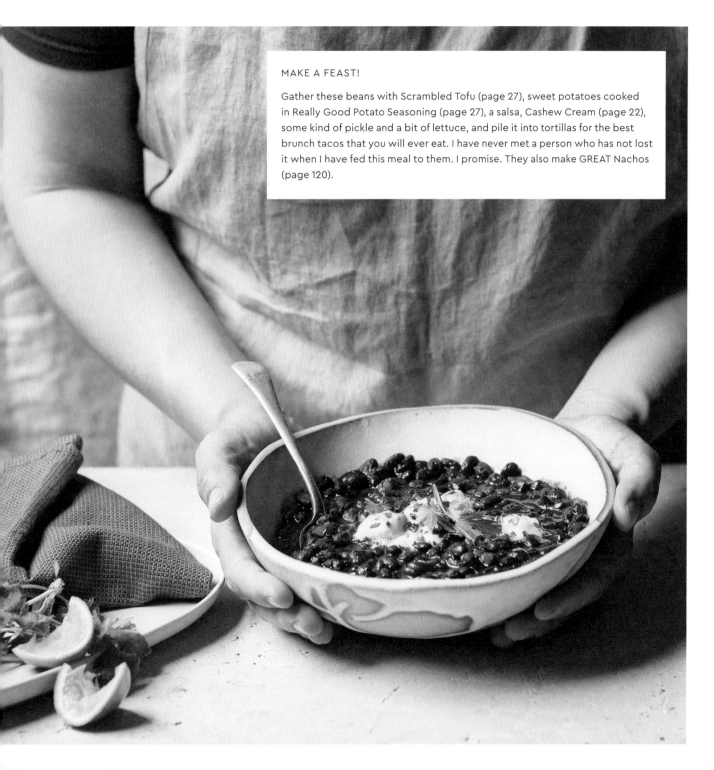

MAKE A FEAST!

Gather these beans with Scrambled Tofu (page 27), sweet potatoes cooked in Really Good Potato Seasoning (page 27), a salsa, Cashew Cream (page 22), some kind of pickle and a bit of lettuce, and pile it into tortillas for the best brunch tacos that you will ever eat. I have never met a person who has not lost it when I have fed this meal to them. I promise. They also make GREAT Nachos (page 120).

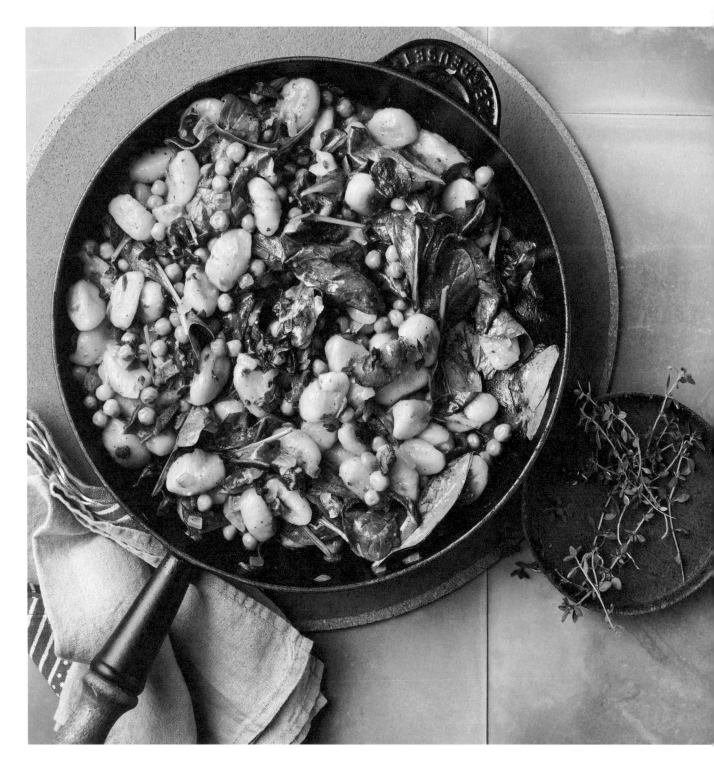

INGREDIENTS
10 g (½ oz) dried wild
    mushrooms
350 ml (12 fl oz/1½ cups)
    boiling water
a few tablespoons of olive oil
1 brown onion, diced
1 × 500 g (1 lb 2 oz) packet
    potato gnocchi
1 large garlic clove,
    finely chopped
1 teaspoon salt
¼ teaspoon ground or
    freshly grated nutmeg
10 sprigs of lemon thyme
150 g (5 oz) frozen peas
100 g (3½ oz) fresh spinach
freshly cracked black pepper
dried chilli (hot pepper) flakes,
    to taste

Mushroom Gnocchi with Peas

Frying gnocchi before adding liquid to the pan has been a one-pot revelation for me that I am so excited to share in this book! Do hunt for the best quality gnocchi you can find, preferably one that is stored in the fridge and not on the shelf (unless you are making at home, in which case, hats off to you). If you can't find wild mushrooms, porcini will do. I don't recommend substituting for shiitakes, which I love but they have a very distinct flavour that doesn't really compliment this dish.

1   Put the mushrooms in a heatproof bowl and cover with the boiling water. Set to one side while you cook the onion and gnocchi.

2   Heat the oil in a large frying pan (skillet) over a medium-high heat. Add the onion and gnocchi and fry for about 10 minutes until the onion is translucent and golden and ever so slightly starting to blacken, using a metal spatula to get all the sticky bits off the base of the pan if you need to.

3   Strain the mushroom soaking liquid and set the mushrooms aside, squeezing any liquid from them into the strained soaking liquid.

4   Add the garlic to the pan and cook for about 1 minute then pour the strained mushroom liquid into the pan. Finely chop the mushrooms and add them to the pan. Add the salt and cook for 10 minutes until the liquid has reduced by half.

5   Add the nutmeg, thyme, peas and spinach. Cook for 2 minutes, then add some pepper and chilli flakes to taste and give it a good stir before spooning into bowls and devouring.

SERVES 4-6

INGREDIENTS

generous glug of olive oil
1 onion, finely chopped
500 g (1 lb 2 oz) brown or button
   mushrooms, cleaned and
   thinly sliced
¼ teaspoon ground or freshly
   grated nutmeg
4 garlic cloves, finely chopped
a few sprigs of fresh lemon thyme
1 litre (34 fl oz/4 cups) vegan
   'chicken' stock
500 ml (17 fl oz/2 cups) soy milk
500 g (1 lb 2 oz) orzo
260 g (9½ oz) frozen spinach
2 tablespoons nutritional yeast
salt and freshly ground
   black pepper

To serve:

8–12 tablespoons spoonfuls of
   Green Pesto (page 21) or
creamy vegan cheese or Cashew
   Cream (page 22) (optional)
dried chilli (hot pepper) flakes,
   to taste
fresh basil leaves

Creamy Mushroom and Spinach Orzo

I am not a fan of having half-used boxes of pasta in my cupboard, so I use an entire box of orzo in this recipe which means it makes a LOT. If you live alone or don't like leftovers, I recommend scaling this recipe down by half.

I make this with lemon thyme because of my love affair of mushrooms with lemon thyme. Do look for it before reaching for something more familar, I promise it's worth it.

1   Heat the oil in large saucepan over a medium heat. Add the onion and mushrooms, a couple of generous pinches of salt and the nutmeg, and cook for at least 20 minutes until the mushrooms have released all their liquid and the onions are soft and golden. Add the garlic and lemon thyme and cook for a minute, then add the stock and soy milk. Bring to the boil and add the orzo. Cook for 8 minutes (or according to the orzo packet instructions), adding the frozen spinach for the final 4 minutes of cooking time, stirring frequently to incorporate the spinach into the dish.

2   Remove from the heat, stir in the nutritional yeast, and season to taste with salt and pepper.

3   Serve the mushroom and spinach orzo in warm bowls, topped with a spoonful of pesto or cream cheese, then scatter with chilli flakes and basil leaves.

4   This dish is best eaten fresh, but leftovers can be stored in the refrigerator for a couple of days and reheated before serving.

> TIP: This dish packs a good protein punch but if you are looking for a boost, add a tin of lentils at any stage during cooking or a tin of cannelini (white) beans when cooking the mushrooms so they break down and get all creamy.

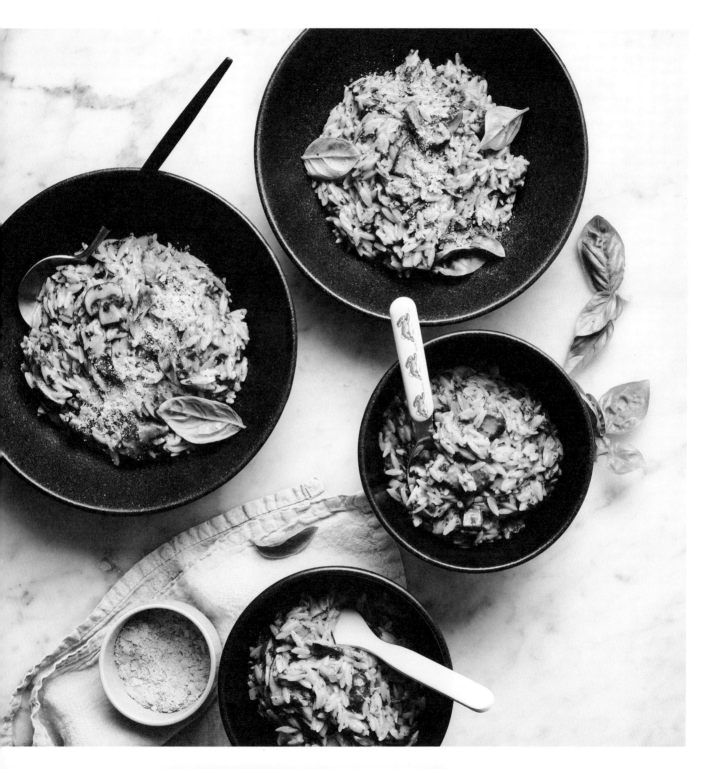

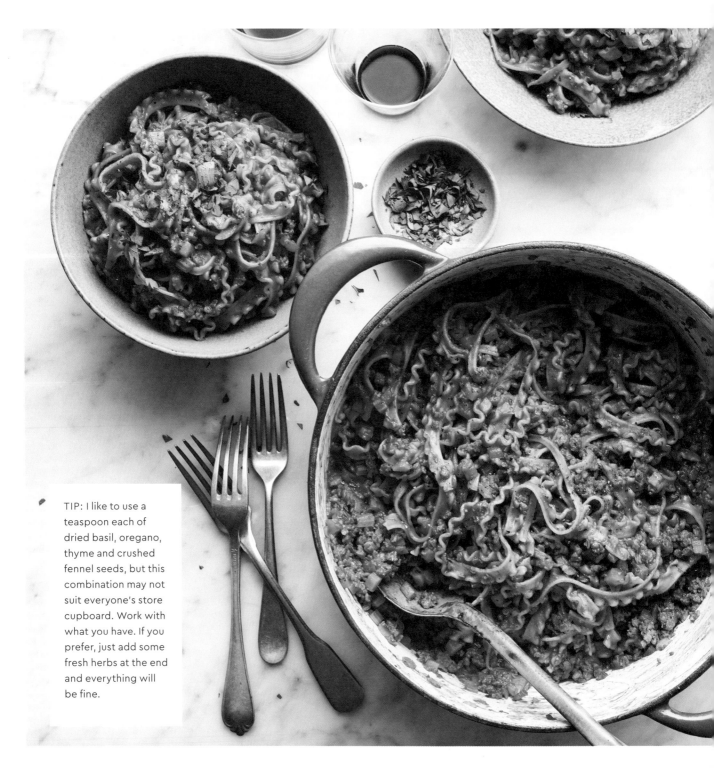

TIP: I like to use a teaspoon each of dried basil, oregano, thyme and crushed fennel seeds, but this combination may not suit everyone's store cupboard. Work with what you have. If you prefer, just add some fresh herbs at the end and everything will be fine.

INGREDIENTS

a very generous glug of olive oil
1 brown onion, very finely
    chopped
2 celery stalks, very finely
    chopped
2 carrots, very finely chopped
400 g (14 oz) vegan mince meat
60 g (2 oz/¼ cup) tomato purée
    (paste)
3–4 garlic cloves, finely chopped
120 ml (4 fl oz/½ cup) red wine
690 g (1 lb 9 oz) jar passata
    (sieved tomatoes)
1 litre (34 fl oz/4 cups) veggie
    stock or vegan 'chicken'
    or 'beef' stock
1 generous teaspoon salt
1 teaspoon sugar
500 g (1 lb 2 oz) dried fettuccine
generous amount of herbs
    (fresh or dried) – see Tip
salt and freshly ground
    black pepper

To serve:

good-quality vegan feta or
    other soft cheese (optional)
fresh herbs such as basil, parsley
    or oregano (optional)
nutritional yeast (optional),
    to taste
dried chilli (hot pepper) flakes,
    to taste

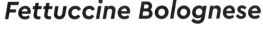

Fettuccine Bolognese

This recipe is more about technique than anything, as how it tastes will ultimately depend on which specific brand of vegan mince meat, type of wine and selection of herbs you use. With that in mind, taste, taste, taste as you go and adjust seasonings as necessary.

As with traditional Bolognese, I would not recommend serving without some kind of 'cheese'. I prefer to go the creamy route, with dollops of vegan cream cheese or chevre melted on top and then stirred in before eating, otherwise use my Sprinkles recipe on page 26.

1   Heat the oil in a large saucepan over a medium-high heat, add the onion, celery and carrots and cook for a good 5–10 minutes until the veggies are soft and starting to turn ever so slightly brown. Add the mince meat and use a wooden spoon to break it up into smaller pieces, add the garlic and cook for a couple of minutes, then add the tomato purée and cook for a couple of minutes, stirring it into the mince. Add the wine and let it cook for a few minutes (until it no longer smells pungent), then add the passata, stock, salt and sugar. Bring to the boil and add the fettuccine and dried herbs (if using). Gently coerce the fettuccine into the sauce, and cook according to the pasta packet instructions, stirring every now and again to make sure nothing is sticking to the bottom of the pan.

2   When the pasta is cooked, remove the pan from the heat, give everything a good stir and cover the pan with a lid. It should still be a little soupy at this stage, but have faith! Allow it to sit for 10 minutes, then remove the lid to reveal a delicious, silky, perfect Bolognese. Taste, season with salt and pepper if necessary, and serve, topped with something creamy, fresh herbs, nutritional yeast (if using) and chilli flakes.

3   Leftover Bolognese will keep well in the refrigerator for up to 4 days. Reheat before serving.

INGREDIENTS

360 g (12½ oz/2 cups) dried
   broad (fava) beans
2 teaspoons bicarbonate of soda
   (baking soda)
generous glug of olive oil
1 brown onion, diced
3–5 garlic cloves, finely chopped
3 dried bay leaves
2 litres (70 fl oz/8 cups) water
2 teaspoons salt

To serve the Berlin way:
fresh flatbread
chopped tomato
chopped onion
chopped cucumber
parsley
olives
pickles

Ful Medames

Andy and I were addicted to this style of Ful that we used to get it as a late breakfast from an Imbiss in Berlin, where there was always this simple but distinctively flavoured broad (fava) bean stew bubbling away in a large pot. They served it to us alongside a plate piled high with raw onion, tomato, lemon, parsley, pickles and olives, and a plastic bag full of flatbread, which is how we now enjoy it at home in Melbourne.

1 Put the broad beans and bicarbonate of soda in a bowl of water and stir to dissolve the soda. Soak the dried beans overnight or for at least 6–8 hours. Drain and rinse before using.

2 Heat the oil in a large saucepan over a high heat, add the onion and cook, stirring, for about 5 minutes until it starts to brown, then add the garlic and bay leaves. Let the garlic and bay sizzle for a minute then add the drained beans and the water. Bring to the boil, reduce the heat and simmer uncovered for 30 minutes – the beans should be starting to soften and will squish easily on the side of the pan. If the skins of the beans still feel a little tough, add a pinch of bicarbonate of soda. Add the salt and use a potato masher to mash some of them in the pan until the liquid thickens a bit. Cook for another 20–30 minutes, so the liquid reduces and the mixture becomes smooth and creamy.

3 Serve the ful medames with flatbread and Berlin-style toppings, or allow to cool and pop in the refrigerator for reheating later. The ful medames will keep in the refrigerator for up to 4 days, but the mixture will thicken when cooled, so when reheating, add water to thin it out a little and get a nice creamy consistency.

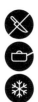

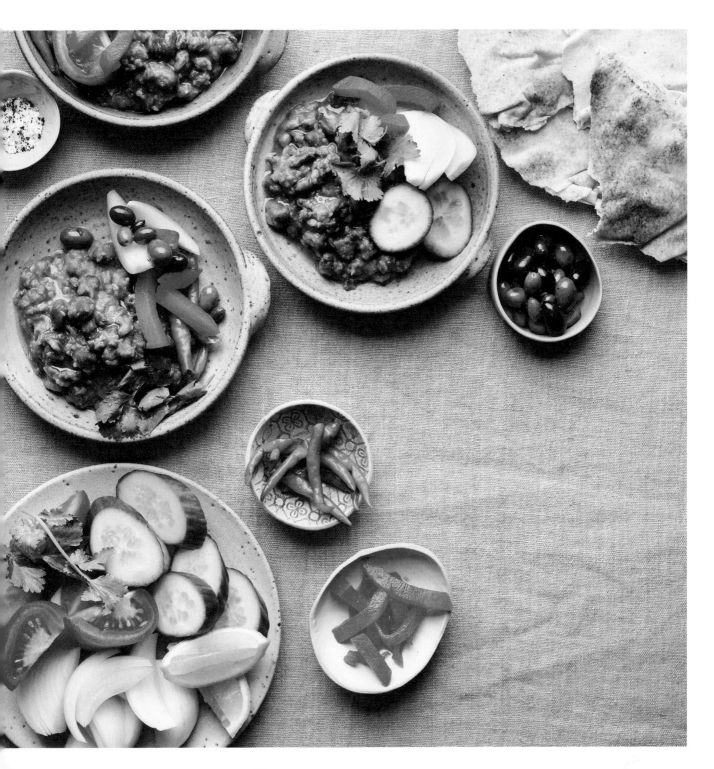

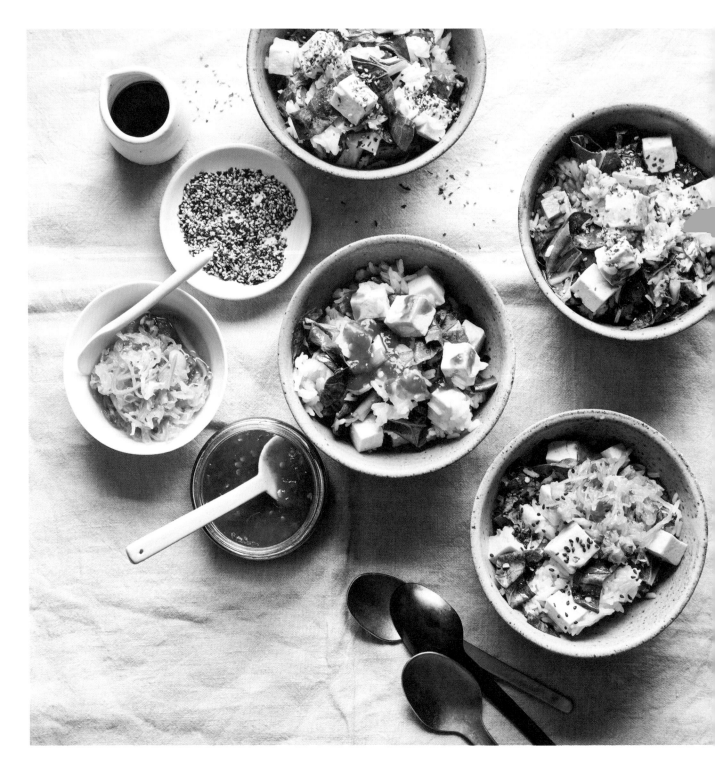

INGREDIENTS

3 tablespoons toasted sesame oil
thumb-size piece of fresh ginger,
    peeled and cut into matchsticks
    or minced
2 garlic cloves, finely minced
400 g (14 oz/2 cups) jasmine rice
400–500 g (14 oz–1 lb 2 oz) firm
    tofu, drained, pressed and cut
    into 1 cm (½ in) cubes
1 litre (34 fl oz/4 cups) vegan
    'chicken' stock
1–2 bunches of pak choi
    (bok choi), choi sum or any
    other kind of Chinese cabbage

CONDIMENTS

Always:
tamari or soy sauce
sambal oelek
furikake or Sesame Seaweed
    Salt Blend (page 26)

Sometimes:
toasted sesame oil
kimchi
toasted sesame seeds
    (if not using furikake)
1 ripe avocado, peeled and sliced
chilli oil or sriracha sauce
    (if not using sambal oelek)

Ginger Jasmine Rice

This dish is hands down the recipe I've cooked most from this book. It's simple, comforting, moreish and one of those dishes that once cooking, basically takes care of itself. Andy loves it, my kids love it, and the leftovers make THE best savoury breakfast.

I always serve it spooned into bowls with an array of condiments at the table for us to help ourselves to, depending on our cravings that day.

1   Heat the sesame oil in a large saucepan over a medium heat. Add the ginger and garlic and cook for about 2 minutes until fragrant. Add the rice and cook, stirring constantly for a couple of minutes, then add the tofu and stock. Cover, bring to the boil then lower the heat and simmer for 18 minutes.

2   While the rice is cooking, cut the greens into roughly 1 cm (½ in)-thick slices, discarding the base. Place in a large bowl and cover with cold water. Agitate the water and leaves a little then transfer the leaves to a colander: this is essential to get all the sandy, gritty bits out. Repeat this step if you're not sure you've removed it all.

3   Once the rice has cooked for 18 minutes, add the drained greens to the pan – just placing it on top of the rice. Cook for a further 2 minutes. Remove from the heat, give everything a stir, then cover and allow to sit for another 10 minutes while you gather your condiments and avocado (if using).

4   Spoon the rice into bowls, top with your favourite condiments and enjoy. Leftovers can be stored in an airtight container in the refrigerator for up to 3 days.

INGREDIENTS

3 tablespoons olive oil
1 onion, finely chopped
2–3 carrots, finely chopped
2–3 celery stalks, finely chopped
stalks from a bunch of fresh
    coriander (cilantro), finely
    chopped (keep the leaves
    to serve)
1 heaped teaspoon ground
    coriander
1 heaped teaspoon ground cumin
3 garlic cloves, finely chopped
2 × 400 g (14 oz) tins black beans
    (or 3 cups of cooked beans)
500 ml (17 fl oz/2 cups) vegan
    'chicken' stock (I use a bouillon
    cube here)
1 heaped teaspoon sweet
    smoked paprika
1 teaspoon salt

To serve:
good-quality salted, organic
    corn chips
4–8 tablespoons vegan sour
    cream or Cashew Cream
    (page 22)
1 ripe avocado, peeled and diced
dried chilli (hot pepper) flakes,
    to taste
1 lime, halved

Black Bean Soup

I've already spoken of my love for cooking black beans from scratch, however I wanted to include a recipe in this book that calls on tinned beans for those times when you want a yum comfort meal in a pinch.

If you have precooked black beans at home, simply swap the tinned beans for three cups of cooked beans. You can also use dried black beans with this recipe if you have a little more time, see my Beloved Black Beans recipe (page 74) and adapt the method of this recipe to suit.

1   Heat the oil in a large saucepan over a medium heat. Add the onion, carrot and celery and cook for at least 10 minutes until the vegetables have softened and are starting to brown. Add the coriander stalks, spices and garlic. Cook for another minute or two, until fragrant, then add the tinned beans and their liquid, stock, paprika and salt. Increase the heat to high, cover and bring to the boil, then reduce the heat and simmer for 10–20 minutes or until the carrots are soft and tender.

2   Enjoy the soup as it is, or purée half of it to give it a thicker, creamier texture. Both ways are delish.

3   To serve, crush a handful of corn chips into the bottom of each serving bowl. Ladle the soup over the top and top with sour cream or cashew cream, a few additional crushed corn chips, diced avocado, chilli flakes, the reserved coriander leaves and a squeeze of fresh lime.

4   Leftovers will keep well in the refrigerator for up to 3–4 days.

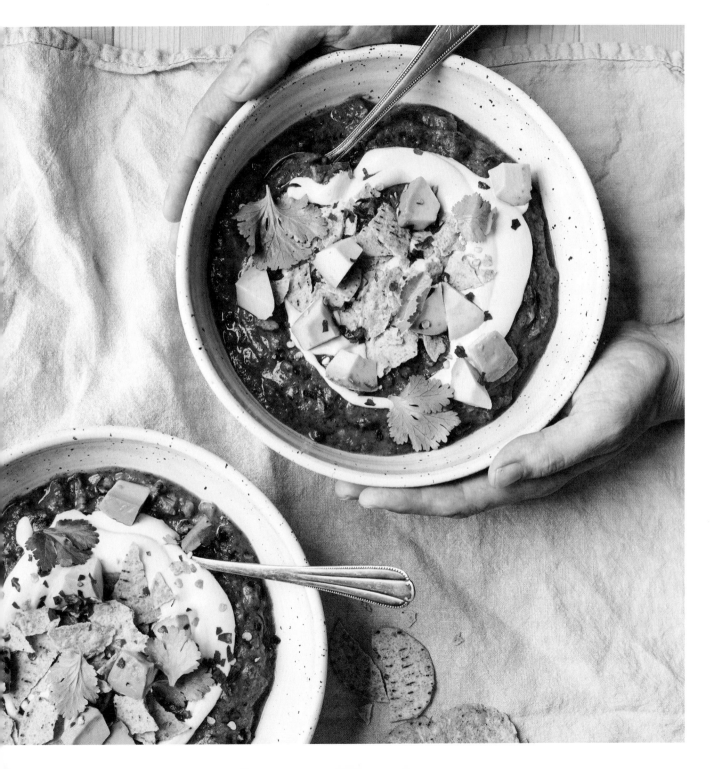

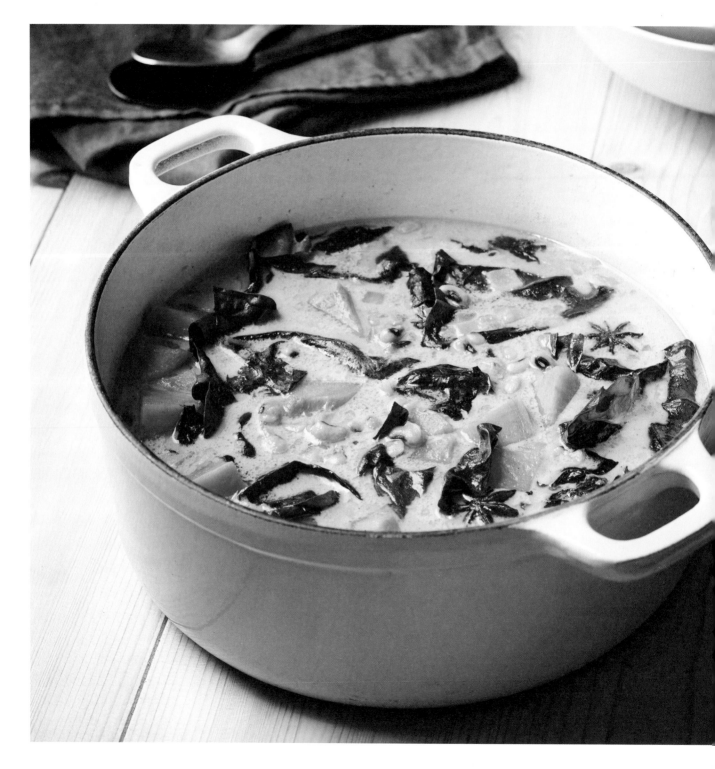

INGREDIENTS

2 tablespoons coconut oil

1 onion, diced

thumb-size piece of fresh ginger, peeled and cut into matchsticks

2 garlic cloves, crushed (minced)

1 tablespoon curry powder

2 star anise

2 × 400 g (14 oz) tins black-eyed beans (peas), drained and rinsed

1 large sweet potato, peeled and cut into bite-size chunks

400 ml (14 fl oz) tin coconut milk

1 litre (34 fl oz/4 cups) vegan 'chicken' stock

a bunch of chard (about 12 large leaves), stems removed and leaves cut or torn into bite-size pieces

salt and freshly ground black pepper (optional)

bread, rice, roti or quinoa, to serve (optional)

For toppings (optional):

handful of fresh coriander (cilantro), leaves picked

dried chilli (hot pepper) flakes, to taste

Golden Black-eyed Beans

I've been making curries like this since my uni days. Back then, I used to put as many vegetables as possible into a curry; however, these days I prefer simpler versions, using just two or three different veggies. This version uses black-eyed beans for protein, sweet potato for carbs and healthy starches, and greens for iron and fibre.

It is filling and moreish on its own but equally as satisfying with homemade bread, roti, rice or quinoa if you wish to bulk it up a little.

1   Heat the coconut oil in a large casserole pot (Dutch oven) or saucepan over a medium-high heat, add the onion and ginger and cook for about 5 minutes, until the onion is translucent and ever so slightly starting to brown. Add the garlic, curry powder and star anise and cook, stirring constantly, for 1–2 minutes until the curry powder is fragrant. Then add the black-eyed beans, sweet potato, coconut milk and stock. Bring to the boil, reduce the heat and simmer uncovered for 20 minutes. Check the sweet potato and once it's tender enough to be easily pierced with a fork, add the chard and cook for 1 minute.

2   Taste and season with salt or pepper if necessary (the stock might make it salty enough not to need additional seasoning) and remove the star anise. Serve immediately, either alone or with bread, rice, roti or quinoa, topped with coriander and chilli flakes (if using).

3   Leftovers will keep well in the refrigerator for up to 4 days.

> TIP: If you can't find tinned black-eyed peas, use chickpeas instead.

INGREDIENTS
200 g (7 oz/1 cup) mung dal
200 g (7 oz/1 cup) basmati rice
3 tablespoons coconut oil
1 onion, diced (optional)
thumb-size piece of fresh ginger,
    peeled and finely minced
3 garlic cloves, finely minced
2-3 teaspoons salt
500 g (1 lb 2 oz) diced seasonal
    veggies, such as pumpkin, sweet
    potato, cauliflower, green beans,
    etc.
1.2-1.4 litres (40-48 fl oz/4¾-6 cups)
    water
juice of 1 lemon
fresh coriander (cilantro),
    to garnish
chutney of choice, to serve

For the spice mix:
1 heaped tablespoon cumin seeds
1 heaped tablespoon coriander seeds
1 heaped tablespoon ground turmeric
1 heaped tablespoon fennel seeds
1 teaspoon yellow mustard seeds
1 teaspoon ground fenugreek
½ teaspoon freshly ground
    black pepper
½ teaspoon asafoetida
½ teaspoon ground cinnamon
sprig of curry leaves

Kitchadee

Kitchadee is a healing ayurvedic dish that is mild in flavour, warming and nutritious, and is eaten on its own for breakfast lunch and dinner a few days in a row when the digestive system needs a pause and reset. I don't have the discipline to eat the same thing for that many meals in a row, but I adore this recipe for its simplicity. Serve with a good-quality Indian chutney if you wish to add tang and texture.

Don't fret if you don't have all the spices, so long as you have cumin, coriander, turmeric and if possible, curry leaves, it will be delicious.

1   Soak the mung dal and basmati rice in a large bowl of cold water overnight, or rinse it in a bowl of water, swishing it to remove the starch, draining and repeating until the water is clear.

2   Combine the spices in a small cup so you have them all together in one place (so they won't burn while you are fiddling around with the spice jars).

3   Warm the coconut oil in a large saucepan over a medium-high heat. Add the onion (if using) and ginger and cook for about 5 minutes, until the onion is translucent, then add the garlic, spice mix and salt, and cook for a minute before adding the drained mung dal and rice. Fry for a minute, then add the veggies and water, stir, and bring to the boil. Reduce the heat to low and simmer for 40 minutes, without removing the lid or stirring the contents. (Tricky, I know, but this is the key to well-cooked rice.)

4   Remove from heat and stir. If you would prefer a more soup-like consistency, add another 250 ml (8½ fl oz/1 cup) of water, stir and then set aside, covered, for 10 minutes.

5   Spoon the kitchadee into bowls, squeeze over the lemon juice, then top with coriander and chutney.

6   Leftovers will keep well in the refrigerator for a couple of days.

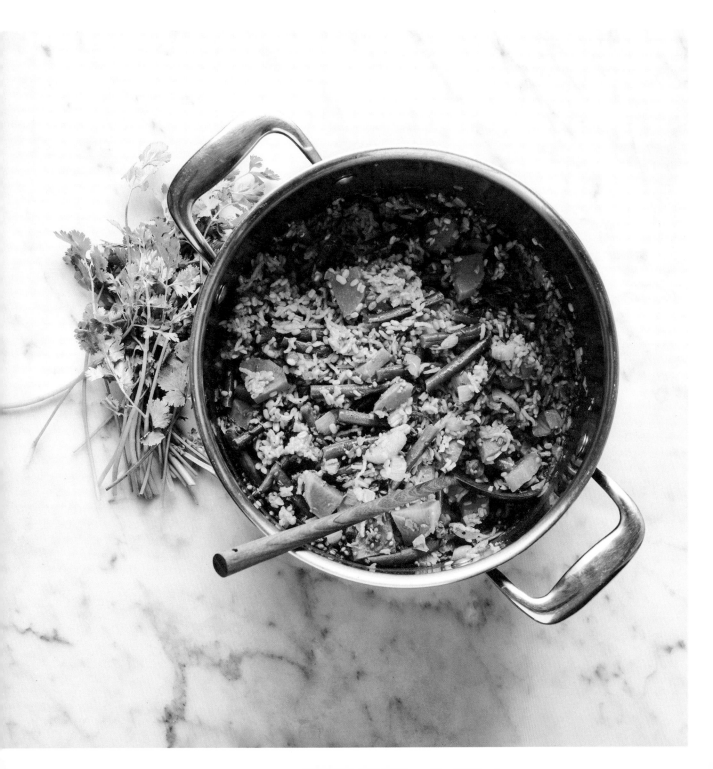

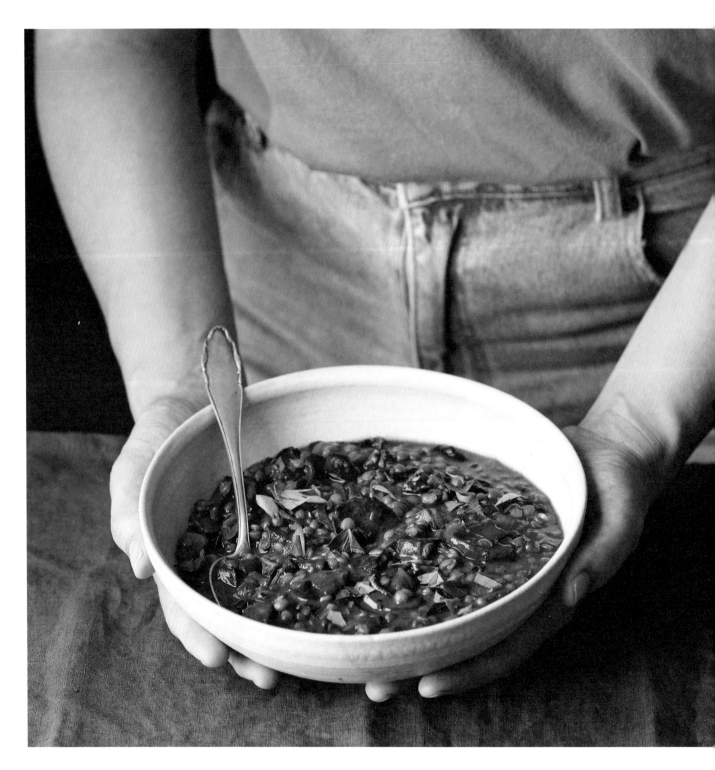

INGREDIENTS

185 g (6½ oz/1 cup) French Green (Puy) lentils, soaked overnight
25 g (¾ oz) dried porcini or forest mushrooms
1 litre (34 fl oz/4 cups) boiling water
generous glug of olive oil
1 large brown onion, diced
500 g (1 lb 2 oz) fresh mushrooms, cleaned, then half cut into small pieces, half sliced
4 tablespoons plain (all-purpose) flour
3 large or 5 small garlic cloves, finely diced
60 g (2 oz/¼ cup) tomato purée (paste)
120 ml (4 fl oz/½ cup) white wine
400 ml (14 fl oz) tin coconut milk
1 teaspoon sweet smoked paprika
½ teaspoon ground nutmeg
dried chilli (hot pepper) flakes, to taste (optional)
salt and freshly ground black pepper
handful of fresh parsley, roughly chopped (optional)

Mushroom and Lentil Stew

A rich, hearty and flavoursome stew with a million ways you can serve it, this dish never fails to hit the spot.

1   Soak the lentils in a large bowl of cold water overnight or for at least 6–8 hours. A quick soak also works, if you're short on time – simply put the lentils in a heatproof bowl, cover them with boiling water and allow to sit for about 1 hour, until ready to cook.

2   Put the dried mushrooms in a heatproof bowl, cover with the boiling water and allow to sit for at least 1 hour.

3   Heat the olive oil in a large saucepan over a medium-high heat, add the onion and cook for about 5 minutes, until it is translucent and ever so slightly starting to brown. Add the chopped mushrooms with a generous pinch of salt and cook for a good 10–15 minutes, until they have drastically reduced in size and all of the liquid they release has evaporated. Don't rush this step – use the time to tend to other kitchen duties.

4   Add the flour, garlic and tomato purée and cook, stirring constantly, for a couple of minutes and then add the wine and cook for a couple minutes more.

5   Drain the lentils and add these to the pan with 2 teaspoons of salt and the coconut milk, as well as the strained liquid from soaking the mushrooms. Finely chop the soaked mushrooms and add these to the pan too, along with the paprika, nutmeg and black pepper and chilli flakes to taste (if using). Increase the heat to high and cook uncovered for 15–20 minutes, until you can easily squish the lentils on the side of the pan with a wooden spoon. Remove from the heat, sprinkle with parsley and serve it any which way your heart desires. My favourite ways with bread (of course), over a baked potato or sweet potato, as a pie filling with flaky pastry, topped with mashed potato as a shepherd's pie, alongside a salad, and on top of pasta.

6   Leftovers will keep well in the refrigerator for up to 4 days.

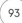

INGREDIENTS

10 g (½ oz) dried porcini
    mushrooms
1 litre (34 fl oz/4 cups) boiling
    water
good glug of olive oil
1 onion, diced
1 leek, white part halved
    lengthways and thinly sliced
1 celery stalk, finely chopped
1 carrot, finely chopped
3 small beetroot (beets)
    (about 300 g/10½ oz), peeled,
    2 finely chopped and 1 grated
3 large or 5 small garlic cloves,
    finely chopped
1 teaspoon caraway seeds
1 teaspoon salt
10 baby potatoes (about 300 g/
    10½ oz), quartered
¼ small cabbage, thinly sliced
1 teaspoon sugar
2 tablespoons sauerkraut juice
    or apple cider vinegar
freshly ground black pepper

To serve:

4 tablespoons good-quality
    vegan sour cream
4 tablespoons chopped dill fronds

Borscht

Borscht is an Eastern European beetroot soup that will forever remind me of my first Christmas in Berlin. Traditionally you would use the mushrooms from the stock as a filling for dumplings that you cook in the soup, but in the spirit of one-pot cooking we are adding them straight into the soup instead.

1   Put the dried porcini mushrooms in a large heatproof bowl and pour over the boiling water. Allow to sit while you prepare the other ingredients.

2   Heat the oil in a large saucepan over a medium-high heat. Add the onion, leek, celery and carrot and sauté for 5–10 minutes until the onion and leek begin to turn ever so slightly brown. Add the chopped and grated beetroot, garlic and caraway seeds, stir for a couple of minutes, then add the water from the mushrooms and the salt. Increase the heat to high.

3   Squeeze any excess water from the soaked mushrooms, finely chop, then add them to the pan, along with the potatoes, cabbage, sugar, sauerkraut juice or vinegar, and black pepper to taste. Cook for 20–30 minutes, until the beetroot and potato are tender. You may need to add another cup of boiling water if the borscht is getting rather thick.

4   Remove from the heat, spoon into bowls and top with vegan sour cream and dill. The soup will keep well in an airtight container in the refrigerator for up to 4 days.

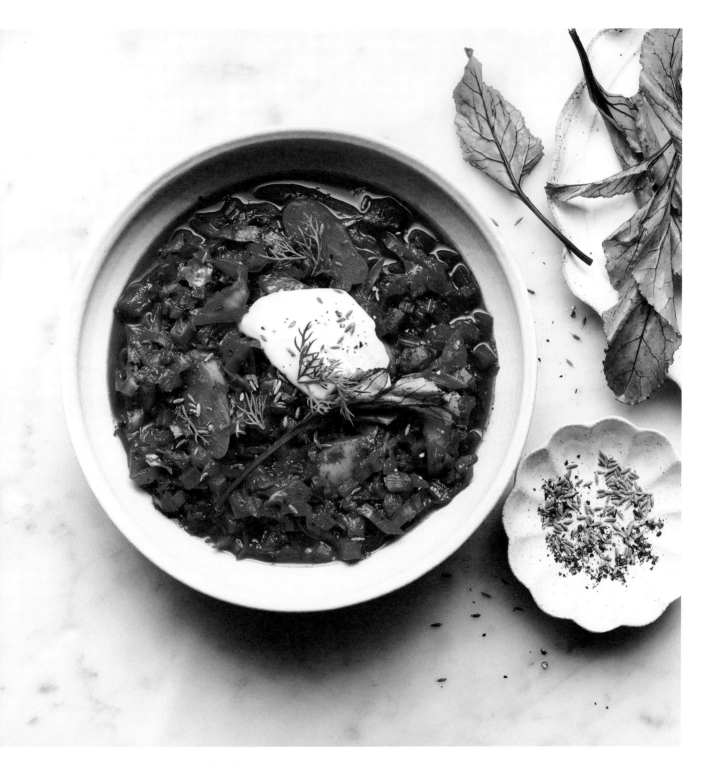

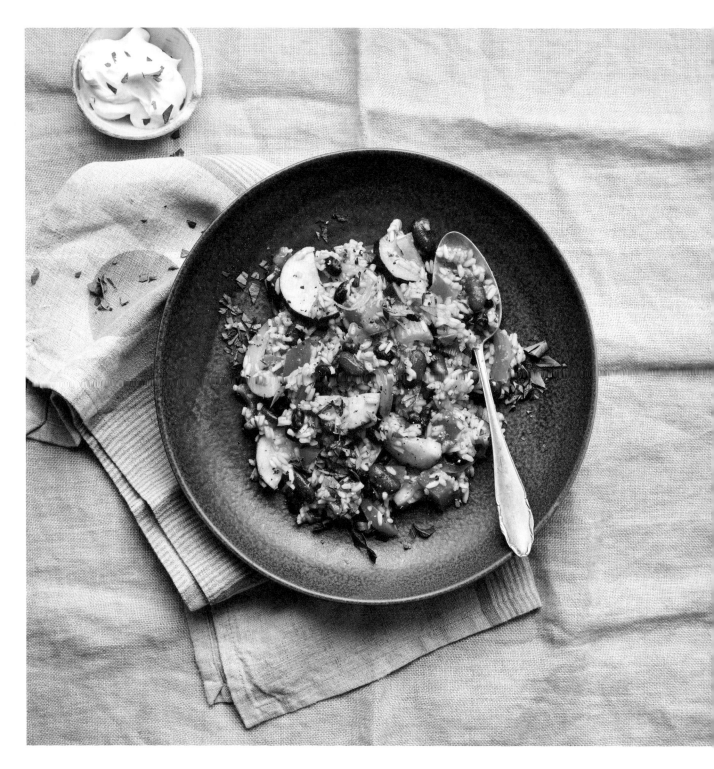

SERVES 4-6

INGREDIENTS

generous glug of olive oil

1 large red onion, cut into thin wedges

2 celery stalks, thinly sliced

1 red (bell) pepper, seeded and diced

1 courgette (zucchini), halved
   lengthways and cut into half-moons

300 g (10½ oz/1½ cups) long-grain
   white rice, rinsed

750 ml (25 fl oz/3 cups) veggie
   stock or vegan 'chicken' stock

400 g (14 oz) tin chopped tomatoes

400 g (14 oz) tin black beans, drained

400 g (14 oz) tin kidney beans, drained
   and rinsed

handful of fresh parsley leaves, finely
   chopped, plus extra to garnish

plain coconut or soy yoghurt,
   to serve

For the spice mix:

2 bay leaves

1 teaspoon salt

1 teaspoon dried thyme

1 teaspoon sweet smoked paprika

½ teaspoon celery seed

½ teaspoon onion powder

½ teaspoon garlic powder

½ teaspoon English mustard powder

½ teaspoon fennel seeds

½ teaspoon freshly cracked
   black pepper

Pa's Jambalaya

My father-in-law is an excellent cook and this is one of my favourite recipes of his. He makes it in a paella pan on the BBQ when he needs to feed the whole fam and it's too hot to cook inside, but a large frying pan (skillet) on the indoor hob works just as well.

1   Put all the spice mix ingredients in a small cup or ramekin and set aside. (This will prevent them burning while you search for/add the other ones.)

2   Heat the oil in a large, high-edged frying pan (skillet) over a medium-high heat. Add the onion wedges and cook for about 3 minutes or until starting to soften. Next, add the celery and red pepper and cook for about 5 minutes, stirring frequently, then add the courgette and cook for a couple of minutes.

3   Add all the spices and cook for a minute or so, until fragrant, then stir in the rice, coating it in the spices and oil. Add the stock, bring to the boil, reduce the heat and simmer uncovered for 10 minutes.

4   Add the tomatoes and both types of beans and cook for a further 5–10 minutes, until the rice is al dente. Remove from the heat and allow to sit, covered, for 5 more minutes before stirring in the parsley and spooning into bowls. Top with yoghurt and extra parsley leaves.

5   Leftovers will keep well in the refrigerator for up to 4 days and freeze beautifully too.

INGREDIENTS
250 g (9 oz) pasta –
    any shape is fine
1 small head of broccoli,
    cut into small florets
olive oil or vegan margarine
nutritional yeast, to taste
dried chilli (hot pepper) flakes,
    to taste
salt and freshly ground
    black pepper

Optional extras:
a few tablespoons of Green
    Pesto (page 21), thinned with
    a bit of pasta cooking water
    if necessary
60 g (2 oz/generous
    ⅓ cup) frozen peas,
    added with the broccoli
    a handful of rocket (arugula)
    or fresh herbs

Pasta Broccoli

A childhood classic revisited. This recipe almost didn't make it into this book because it is so unbelievably simple, it was almost overlooked, despite the fact that I make this for my kids at least five nights per week. Traditionally served with Parmesan, in our house we serve with nutritional yeast, salt, pepper and chilli and it is eaten with gusto, every time.

1   Bring a large saucepan of salted water to a rolling boil. Add the pasta and cook according to the packet instructions, adding the broccoli for the final 5 minutes of cooking time. (The point is for the broccoli to get soft, which is what adds to the comfort-food factor. If you prefer your broccoli crunchy, add it for the final minute only.)

2   Drain the pasta and broccoli and return it to the pan with a generous amount of olive oil or vegan margarine, salt, pepper and nutritional yeast. Stir to combine, so the broccoli starts to ever so slightly break down and coat the pasta. Serve in bowls, topped with additional salt, pepper, nutritional yeast and chilli flakes (if using).

3   You can tweak the recipe, adding any of the optional extras listed, if you like. Leftovers keep in the fridge for up to 3 days.

> TIP: If you are worried about not getting enough protein in your diet, use chickpea (garbanzo) pasta. You may have to shop around as there are some terrible ones out there, but when you do find the perfect chickpea pasta it is more than worth it.

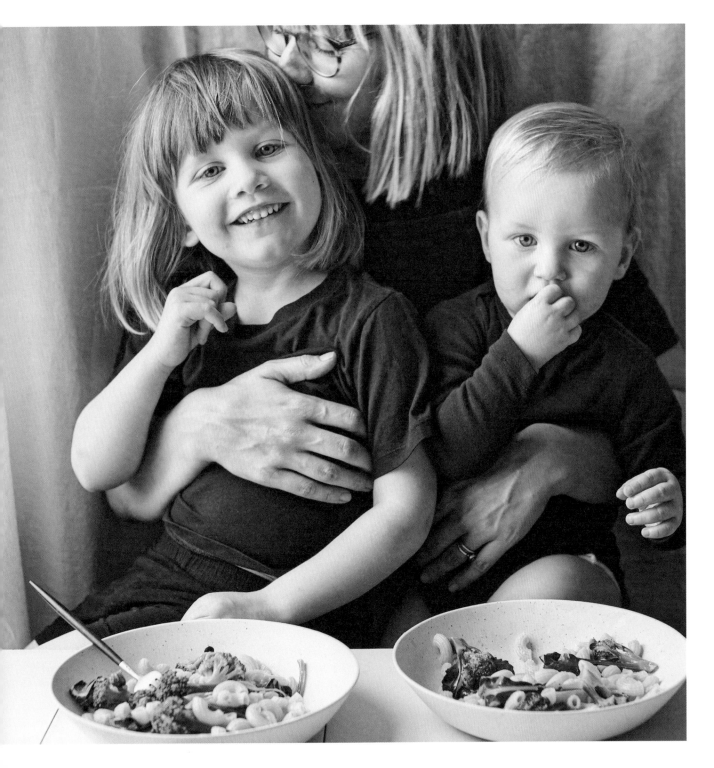

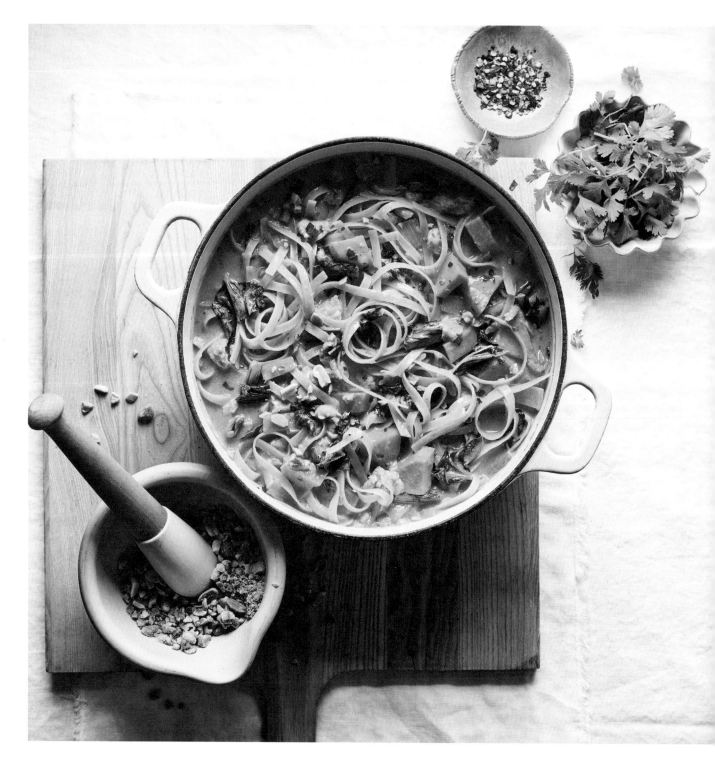

SERVES 4-6

INGREDIENTS

2–3 tablespoons coconut oil
1 onion, diced
thumb-size of fresh ginger,
    peeled and finely minced
3 large garlic cloves, finely minced
4 kaffir lime leaves, torn
1 litre (34 fl oz/4 cups) veggie
    or vegan 'chicken' stock
60 g (2 oz/¼ cup) tomato purée
    (paste)
125 g (4 oz/½ cup) natural peanut
    butter
400 ml (14 fl oz) tin coconut milk
1 large sweet potato (about
    650 g/1 lb 7 oz), peeled and
    cut into bite-size dice
200 g (7 oz) tempeh
big bunch of Chinese broccoli,
    sliced
200 g (7 oz) packet pad Thai
    (flat rice) noodles

To garnish:
handful of fresh coriander
    (cilantro) leaves
dried chilli (hot pepper) flakes
crushed roasted peanuts

Peanut Noodles

*Of all the recipes in this book, this one has the most hectic ingredients
list. I know it seems odd but you gotta trust me here – the end result is
outrageously good.*

1   Heat the oil in a large saucepan or casserole pot (Dutch oven) over a medium-
    high heat, add the onion and ginger and cook for a good 5–10 minutes, until the
    onion is ever so slightly starting to brown.

2   Add the garlic and kaffir lime leaves and cook, stirring, for a minute. Then add
    the stock, tomato purée and peanut butter and stir until they are well combined.

3   Add the coconut milk and sweet potato, then crumble in the tempeh (rather than
    simply cutting it). Simmer uncovered for 20 minutes or until you can pierce the
    sweet potato easily with a fork.

4   Add the Chinese broccoli and simmer for another couple of minutes, then add
    the noodles and immerse them in the liquid. Remove from heat, cover and allow
    to sit for 5 minutes then check the noodles – they should be soft.

5   Serve in bowls, garnished with coriander, chilli flakes and roasted peanuts.

SERVES 4-6

INGREDIENTS

200 g (7 oz/1 cup) dried beluga
    (black) lentils, washed and
    checked over for any stones
3 tablespoons olive oil
1 onion, finely chopped
1 generous teaspoon ground cumin
1 generous teaspoon ground coriander
2-3 portobello mushrooms
    (about 200 g/7 oz), cleaned
    and cut into bite-size pieces
600 ml (20 fl oz/2½ cups) water
¼ pumpkin or ½ butternut squash
    (approx. 500 g/1 lb 2 oz), seeded
    and coarsely grated
400 g (14 oz) tin chopped tomatoes
400 g (14 oz) tin black beans,
    drained and rinsed
3 garlic cloves, finely chopped
1 generous teaspoon sweet
    smoked paprika
a few handfuls of baby spinach
    (about 200 g/7 oz)
handful of fresh coriander (cilantro),
    finely chopped, plus extra to garnish
salt and freshly ground black pepper

To serve (optional):
baked potato, bread, organic
    corn chips, cooked quinoa, rice,
    burritos, etc.
something creamy and tangy such as
    coconut yoghurt, Cashew Cream
    (page 22) or vegan sour cream
1 ripe avocado, peeled and sliced
fresh chilli or smoked paprika

Pumpkin and Lentil Stew

Like many of my stews this is hearty, filling and unbelievably versatile in the ways it can be served. My favourite is over a baked potato but as with my other stews, cooked grains, bread, pasta and for this one – even corn chips are fair game.

1   Soak the lentils in a bowl of water overnight or for at least 6–8 hours. A quick soak also works, if you're short on time – simply put the lentils in a heatproof bowl, cover them with boiling water and allow to sit for about 1 hour, until ready to cook.

2   Heat the oil in medium saucepan over a medium heat, add the onion and cook for about 5 minutes, until translucent and starting to brown, then add the spices and cook for about 2 minutes until fragrant. Add the mushrooms and a generous couple of pinches of salt, cook for 5 minutes, then add the drained lentils and the fresh water. Stir and increase the heat to high. Add the squash or pumpkin, tomatoes, beans, garlic, paprika and a teaspoon of salt. Once bubbling, reduce the heat to medium and cook uncovered for about 20 minutes until thick and stew-like. Stir in the spinach and coriander and season with black pepper to taste.

3   Serve in bowls, either alone or on top of a baked potato, cooked quinoa, cooked rice or corn chips, topped with something creamy, slices of avocado and fresh or smoked chilli.

4   Leftovers will keep well in the refrigerator for up to 4 days, and it freezes well, too.

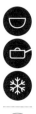

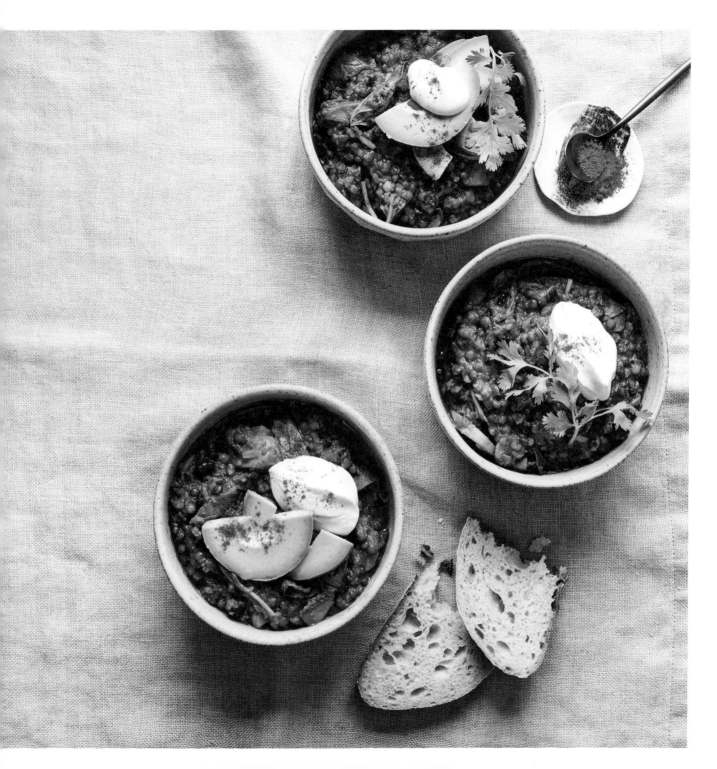

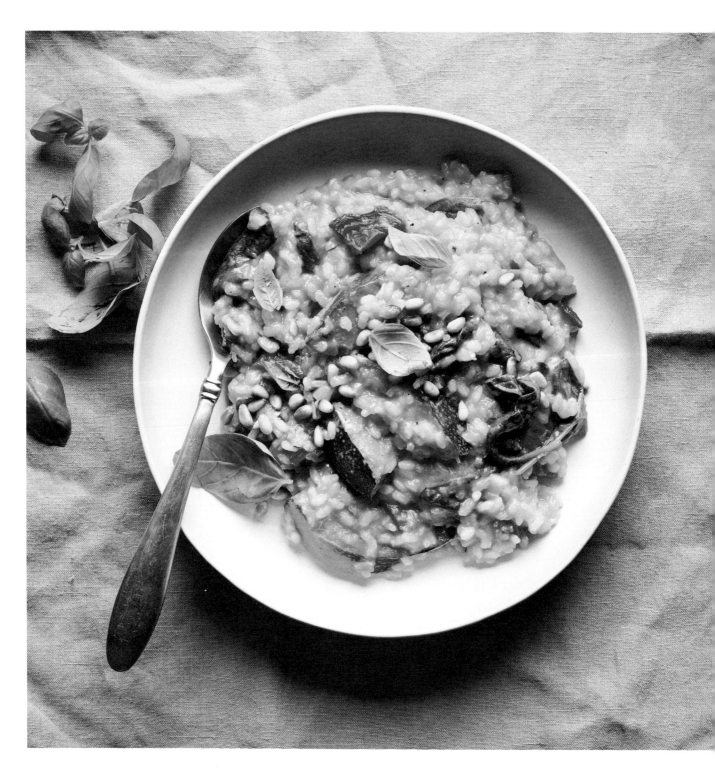

INGREDIENTS

generous glug of olive oil

1 onion, diced

about 500 g (1 lb 2 oz) pumpkin, seeded, and flesh cut into 1 cm (½ in) pieces (leave skin on if possible)

1 litre (34 fl oz/4 cups) veggie stock or vegan 'chicken' stock

300 g (10½ oz/1½ cups) arborio rice

3–5 garlic cloves, finely minced

100 ml (3½ fl oz/scant ½ cup) white wine

3–4 tablespoons nutritional yeast

1 teaspoon salt

a good handful of sundried tomatoes (about 150 g/5 oz), cut into bite-size pieces

a good few handfuls of baby spinach (about 150 g/5 oz)

as much fresh basil as you can get your hands on

lots of freshly cracked black pepper

dried chilli (hot pepper) flakes, to taste (optional)

generous handful of toasted pine nuts, lightly crushed in a mortar and pestle

Pumpkin, Spinach and Sundried Tomato Risotto

This is a recipe from my Berlin dinner party days, which makes it surprising that it never made it into one of my earlier cookbooks. Yet here we are, and I am so glad I waited.

1   Heat the olive oil in a large saucepan over a medium-high heat. Add the onion and pumpkin and cook, stirring every now and again with a wooden spoon, for 20 minutes. It's okay if some of the onion or pumpkin catches to the bottom of the pan – this will come away easily when you add the wine.

2   Boil a kettle full of water and measure out your vegetable stock in a heatproof jug so that you have the hot stock ready to go.

3   Once the onion and pumpkin have been cooking for 20 minutes, add the rice and garlic and cook for 2–3 minutes, stirring constantly. Add the wine and cook, stirring constantly, for another 3–5 minutes, using your wooden spoon to shift any bits that have stuck to the bottom of the pan. Add a cup of hot stock and stir, stir, stir. It is recommended to allow each cup of stock to be absorbed by the rice before adding more, but I have cheated in the past and added all of it so I could join dinner guests in the living room and it was fine! I just made sure everyone knew to give it a stir when walking past. Now that I have kids, it's much the same, and if I'm worried that too much liquid will be absorbed before I can get back to the hob and add the next lot, I plonk it all in and give it a good stir whenever I can. If it's spluttering too much, reduce the heat to medium.

4   After about 30 minutes, the rice should be cooked, the liquid should have all been absorbed, and the pumpkin should be mushy with some chunks remaining. Remove from the heat and add the nutritional yeast, salt, sundried tomatoes, spinach and half the basil and stir until the spinach is wilted. Add plenty of black pepper to taste (and chilli if using).

5   Spoon into warm bowls and top with pine nuts and the rest of the basil.

6   Risotto is best eaten fresh, but you can store leftovers in the refrigerator for up to 4 days, adding a little water when reheating to get it to a silky consistency.

INGREDIENTS

generous glug of olive oil

10–15 big chard leaves

400 g (14 oz) packet vegan Italian
   sausages (or any good-quality,
   yum vegan sausages you can find)

1 red onion, cut into half-moons

3 garlic cloves, finely chopped

2 tablespoons tomato purée (paste)

500 ml (17 fl oz/2 cups) vegan
   'chicken' stock

400 g (14 oz) tin cannellini (white)
   beans, drained and rinsed

dried chilli (hot pepper) flakes,
   to taste

salt and freshly ground
   black pepper

2–3 slices day-old bread, diced,
   to serve

Sausage and White Bean Stew

*Reminiscent of ribollita, this stew is a great way to use up stale bread
and of all my soupy, stewy dishes, it is Andy's fave. Do buy the best quality
vegan sausages you can afford, the extra money is always worth it.*

1   Heat the oil in a large frying pan (skillet) over a medium-high heat. While you are
    waiting for the oil to heat up, remove the woody stems from the chard and cut
    the chard leaves into bite-size pieces. Put the leaves into a large bowl, cover with
    water and allow to sit. Before cooking it, drain off the water and give the leaves a
    shake but don't dry them completely.

2   When the oil is warm, add the sausages to the pan and fry, turning them often,
    for 5–10 minutes until brown and crispy all over. When the sausages are cooked,
    transfer to a paper towel.

3   Add the onion to the pan, with a little extra oil if necessary. Cook for a good
    5–10 minutes, stirring now and again, until they start to turn golden, then add the
    garlic and cook for another minute. Add as much chard as you can fit into the pan
    and cook, tossing and stirring, until it begins to wilt, then make room for the rest
    of the chard and add it to the pan (if you couldn't get it all in in one go).

4   Dissolve the tomato purée in the stock then pour the stock into the pan along
    with the beans.

5   Slice the sausages – which should now be cool enough to touch – into 1 cm
    (½ in) rounds, add them to the stew and cook for another couple of minutes
    until the greens have completely wilted. Remove from the heat and add chill
    flakes, salt and pepper, to taste.

6   Place a handful of diced bread in the bottom of each bowl, ladle the stew over
    top, making sure to get some of the broth so that it pools in the bottom of the
    bowl and can be soaked up by the bread.

7   Leftovers will keep well in the refrigerator for up to 2–3 days.

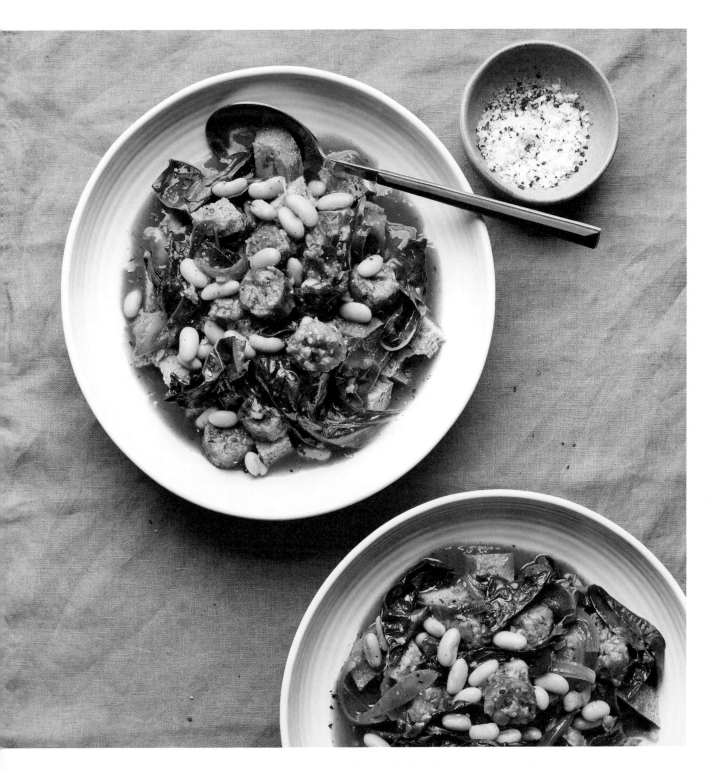

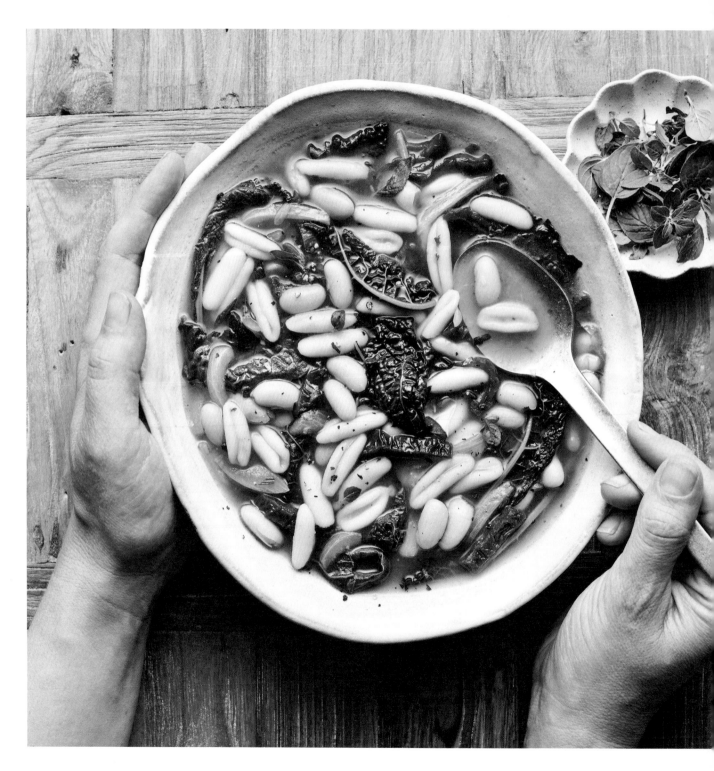

INGREDIENTS
2 tablespoons olive oil
1 red onion, cut into 1 cm (½ in)-
    thick slices
2–3 garlic cloves, finely chopped
heaps of fresh herbs, such as
    rosemary, oregano, lemon
    thyme, sage (not too much),
    and parsley, leaves picked
    and roughly chopped
1 litre (34 fl oz/4 cups) veggie
    stock or vegan 'chicken' stock
1 litre (34 fl oz/4 cups) water
250 g (9 oz) dried soup pasta
    such as orecchiette,
    gnocchiette, mini shells, etc.
2 × 400 g (14 oz) tins cannellini
    (white) beans, drained
    and rinsed
150 g (5 oz/1 cup) sundried
    tomatoes, thinly sliced (get
    the ones not in oil, if possible)
big bunch of Tuscan kale (or *cime
    de rapa* if you get lucky), tough
    stems removed, leaves cut into
    bite-size pieces
juice of ½ lemon
salt and freshly ground
    black pepper
dried chilli (hot pepper) flakes,
    to taste
bread, to serve (optional)

Soupy Pasta Fagioli with Kale

The cover recipe! This humble dish is one of my favourite comfort meals. It was shared with me by a friend many moons ago and has become a mainstay in my home because it is just so good. I use quite an assortment of herbs because I have them all growing in my garden, but don't stress if you can't find them all, it's delicious no matter what combination you use. Likewise with the greens – my neighbour leaves me big bunches of greens all year round, and in the tiny window where she has rapa, I use that in place of the kale.

1   Heat the oil in a large saucepan over a medium heat. Add the onion and cook for about 3 minutes, until it softens. Then add the garlic and herbs and cook for about 1 minute, just until fragrant, stirring to ensure the garlic doesn't burn. Add the stock, water and a teaspoon of salt, cover and bring to the boil.

2   Once the stock is boiling, add the pasta and cook according to the pasta packet instructions, adding the beans, sundried tomatoes and kale for the final 5 minutes of cooking time, stirring every so often to make sure the pasta isn't sticking to the base of the pan.

3   Remove from the heat and allow to sit uncovered for 10 minutes, then add a squeeze of lemon juice, pepper and chilli flakes to taste (and more salt if it needs it).

4   Ladle into bowls and serve with bread if you're a hardcore carb-lover like me.

INGREDIENTS

375 g (13 oz/2 cups) dried French
 green lentils (Puy), washed
3 tablespoons olive oil
1 onion, finely chopped
3 carrots, diced
3 celery stalks, finely chopped
3 large or 5 small garlic cloves,
 finely chopped
2 tablespoon cumin seeds
1 teaspoon ground fenugreek
 (optional)
1 litre (34 fl oz/4 cups) veggie
 stock
500 ml (17 fl oz/2 cups) water
2 large bunches of kale, chard,
 collard greens or any other
 seasonal greens
salt and freshly ground
 black pepper

To serve (optional):
sauerkraut
bread or cooked quinoa

Super Green Lentil Soup

*I make soup on the hottest of summer days, it's a strange habit of mine.
This one holds the dearest place in my heart because I ate it almost every
day in the summer that followed Jude's birth and found it so nourishing,
I decided to make it a core item in the Nourish Packs that my biz Mama
Goodness delivers around Melbourne every Tuesday.*

1   Soak the lentils in a bowl of water overnight or for at least 6–8 hours. A quick
    soak also works, if you're short on time – simply put the lentils in a heatproof bowl,
    cover them with boiling water and allow to sit for 1 hour until you're ready to cook.

2   Heat the oil in a large saucepan over a medium heat, add the onion and cook
    for a couple of minutes until softened but not browned, then add the carrot and
    celery and cook for another 5–10 minutes until softened and starting to brown.
    Add the garlic, cumin seeds and fenugreek (if using) and cook for about 2 minutes
    until fragrant.

3   Drain the lentils and add them to the pan along with the stock and water. Bring
    to the boil and cook for 20 minutes, or until the lentils squish easily on the side
    of the pan when pressed with a wooden spoon.

4   While the lentils are cooking, prepare your greens. Cut the leaves in half (and half
    again if using very wide leaves), removing tough stems, then cut the leaves into
    2 cm- (¾ in-) wide strips. You basically want to get the greens into bite-size
    pieces. Pop the greens in a large bowl and cover with water to remove any dirt,
    drain and set aside.

5   Once the lentils are cooked, add the greens and cook for another 5–10 minutes,
    then remove from the heat. Season with salt and pepper to taste.

6   I like to serve in bowls, topped with sauerkraut and eaten as is. It's good with
    bread (of course, what isn't?), and also very good served on top of cooked
    quinoa if you happen to have any in the refrigerator or freezer.

7   The soup will keep for up to 5 days in an airtight container in the refrigerator,
    and freezes beautifully.

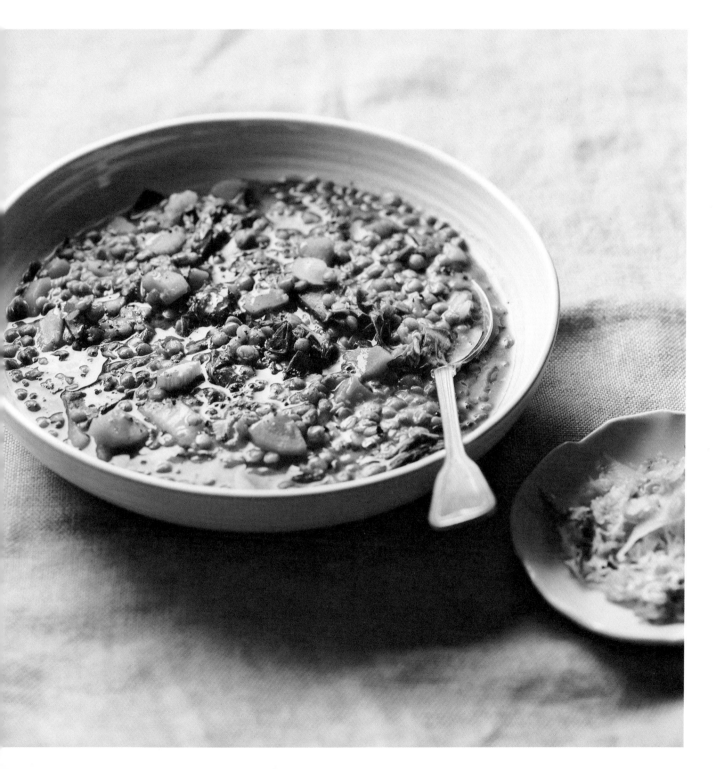

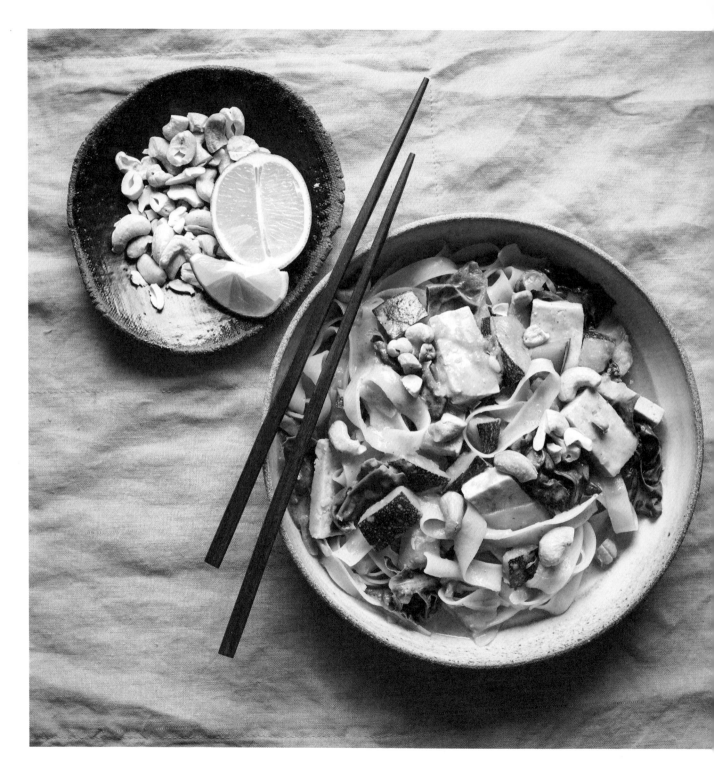

SERVES 4

INGREDIENTS

3 tablespoons coconut oil
1 red onion, sliced
100 g (3½ oz) red curry paste
3–5 garlic cloves, crushed
(minced)
about 400 g (14 oz) pumpkin,
seeded and diced
about 400 g (14 oz) tofu, drained
and pressed, then cut into
bite-size pieces
1 litre (34 fl oz/4 cups) veggie
stock or vegan 'chicken' stock
400 ml (14 fl oz) tin coconut milk
generous bunch of chard, leaves
torn into bite-size pieces
and washed well
salt
200 g (7 oz) pad Thai (flat rice)
noodles

To garnish:
a few handfuls of roasted
cashews, slightly crushed
a handful of fresh coriander
(cilantro) leaves
1 lime, halved (optional)

Thai Red Curry and Pumpkin Noodles

So easy, so yum, so delish, my favourite part about this dish is the way the pumpkin breaks down and becomes a part of the broth, rather than something that is simply floating in it.

1 Heat the coconut oil in a large saucepan over a medium-high heat. Once melted, add the onions and cook for a good 5 minutes, until soft and starting to turn translucent. Add the curry paste and garlic and stir constantly for a minute or so, until the curry paste is fragrant. Add the pumpkin and tofu and cook, stirring, for a couple of minutes, then add the stock and coconut milk. Increase the heat to high, bring to the boil, then reduce the heat to a simmer. Cover and cook, stirring occasionally, for about 20 minutes, or until the pumpkin is almost tender and the edges of the pieces are melding into the soup broth. Add the chard and cook for another 2 minutes, then remove from the heat. Season to taste (if necessary: the stock might make it salty enough).

2 Add the noodles to the pan, nestling them in the broth, then cover and leave for 5 minutes. After 5 minutes, give the noodles a stir and check how well cooked they are: you may need to cover them for another minute or two, depending on the brand of noodle.

3 Ladle the noodles and curried pumpkin into bowls and top with cashews, coriander and a squeeze of lime juice (if using). Enjoy immediately.

4 Leftovers will thicken significantly but it's really delicious the next day (and will keep in the refrigerator for up to 4 days).

INGREDIENTS
generous glug of olive oil
1 onion, finely chopped
4 garlic cloves, finely chopped
2 × 400 g (14 oz) tins chopped
    tomatoes
1 litre (34 fl oz/4 cups) boiling
    water
1 tablespoon sugar
1 teaspoon each of dried basil,
    oregano, celery seeds, sweet
    smoked paprika, fennel
    seeds and dried thyme (or
    2 tablespoons Mama Goodness
    Spice Blend – page 27)
500 g (1 lb 2 oz) dried spaghetti
2 teaspoons salt
heaps of fresh basil
4–6 tablespoons good-quality
    soft or sprinkly vegan cheese,
    to serve

Tomato and Basil Spaghetti

One-pot pasta has revolutionised weeknight cooking but this recipe is so much more than that. It is a base that you can build on with countless variations of vegetable additions and endless types of pasta. My whole family loves it, which is HUGE if you know how resistant our dear Louie is to anything saucy.

If you don't have all of the dried herbs I've listed, swap the water for veggie stock for a flavour boost, and adjust the salt accordingly.

1   Heat the oil in a large saucepan over a medium-high heat, add the onion and garlic and cook for about 5 minutes until soft and starting to brown. Add the chopped tomatoes and simmer for 1 minute, then add the boiling water, sugar and dried herbs, and the spaghetti and salt. Stir to make sure the pasta isn't sticking together or to the base of the pan.

2   Cook for 10 minutes (or according to the pasta packet instructions), until soupy in consistency. Then stir in the basil and set aside, covered, for 10 minutes – it will thicken significantly. Spoon into bowls and top with soft or sprinkly vegan cheese.

OPTIONAL EXTRAS

• Cook mushrooms with the onion and garlic.

• Add one or a few of the following in the final few minutes of cooking: broccoli/frozen spinach/tinned cannellini (white) beans/tinned lentils.

• Stir in at end: olives/pesto (see my Green Pesto on page 21)/fresh spinach.

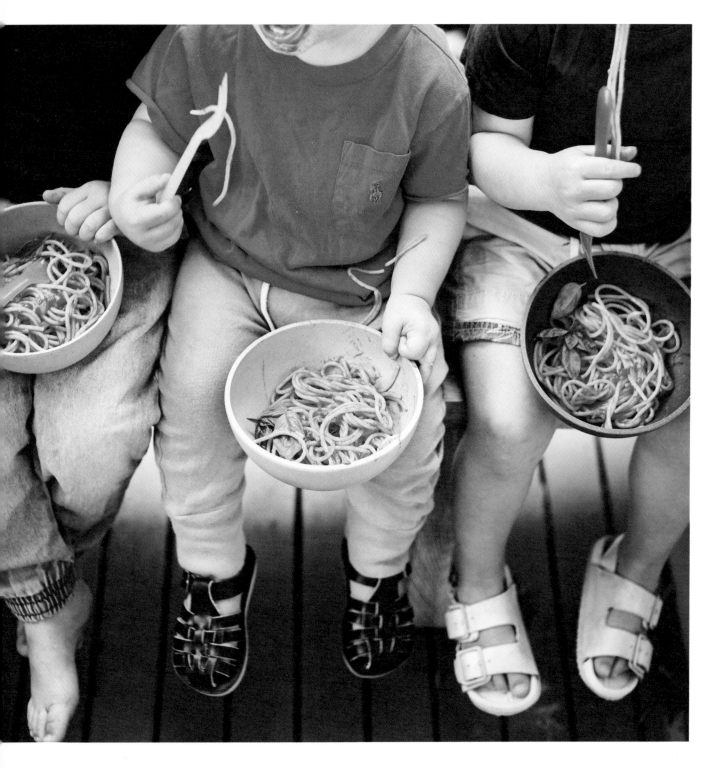

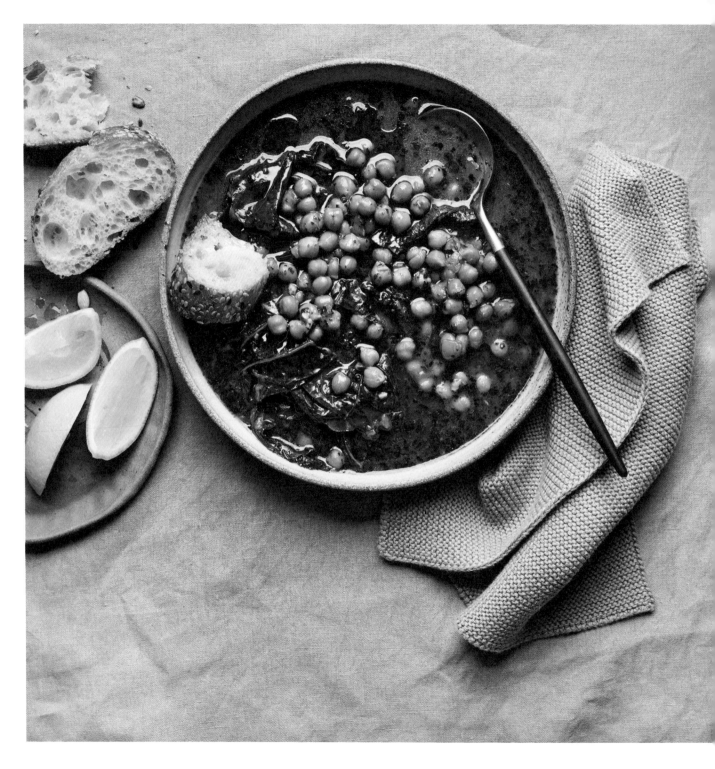

INGREDIENTS

225 g (8 oz/1 cup) dried chickpeas
    (garbanzos)
1 teaspoon bicarbonate of soda
    (baking soda)
1.4 litres (48 fl oz/6 cups) water
2 large red onions, diced
4 garlic cloves, crushed (minced)
10 g (½ oz) dried oregano
½ teaspoon dried thyme
3 large dried bay leaves
2 teaspoons sea salt
1 teaspoon freshly ground
    black pepper
5 tablespoons olive oil,
    plus extra to serve
big bunch of chard, tough stems
    removed, leaves cut into
    large pieces
lemon, to serve

The Village Chickpea Stew

This recipe was shared with me by a dear friend and is now a mainstay in my home. It comes from The Village *– the absolutely stunning and truly heartwarming second cookbook by Matt and Lentil of Grown and Gathered, that explores the key elements of Village living and why they are essential for longevity.*

I've bastardised the original version by making it ready to cook in less than two hours, and by adding chard right at the very end of cooking, which I have in abundance thanks to my adorable neighbour from three doors down.

1   Put the dried chickpeas in a bowl with lots of water and the bicarbonate of soda, stir to dissolve the soda, then leave to soak overnight or for at least 8 hours.

2   Drain and rinse the chickpeas well, then place them in a large saucepan with the water. Cover, bring to the boil, then reduce the heat and simmer, covered, for 1 hour, checking occasionally and skimming off any foam that may have formed on the surface.

3   After 1 hour, the chickpeas should be starting to soften. Add the onions, garlic, oregano, thyme, bay leaves, salt, pepper and olive oil and cook for a further 30 minutes–1 hour, until the chickpeas are delectably soft. Add the chard and stir through for a couple of minutes, until wilted.

4   Serve the stew in bowls, with a drizzle of olive oil and a squeeze of lemon juice, discarding bay leaves as you come across them.

5   The stew will keep in the refrigerator for up to 4 days, or can be frozen.

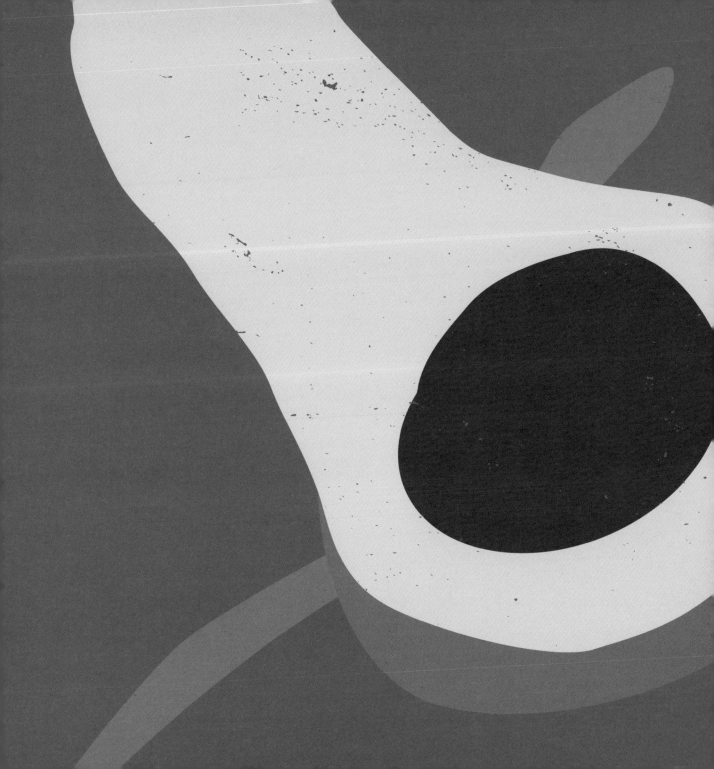

Easy Oven

As mentioned earlier, some of
these recipes dirty a mixing bowl
or glass jug before transferring
contents to the actual cooking
vessel but I promise you, any recipe
that does this is unbelievably
simple in every other way which
I hope you will agree, renders them
a one-pot wonder and worthy
of their place in this book.

INGREDIENTS

a few handfuls of salted
    organic corn chips
260 g (9½ oz/1½ cups) Beloved
    Black Beans (page 74)
    or 400 g (14 oz) tin black beans,
    drained and rinsed (do not
    drain and rinse them if they
    are homemade)
about 330 g (11 oz) good-
    quality jarred Mexican salsa
    (or homemade – see box)
1–2 handfuls of grated cheese
    (vegan or not – it's up to you)
pickled jalapeños or dried chilli
    (hot pepper) flakes, to taste

To serve (optional):

1 ripe avocado, peeled and diced
generous drizzle of Cashew
    Cream (page 22) or vegan
    sour cream
handful of fresh coriander
    (cilantro) leaves

Andy's Nachos

*When left to his own devices for dinner, Andy inevitably makes one
of two things – dad pasta or nachos.*

*You can make these either with my Beloved Black Beans (page 74)
or with tinned ones, however tinned black beans have very little flavour
so I am personally not such a fan of putting them on top of nachos.
Andy usually uses nasty (but delicious) salsa from a jar but if feeding
friends for his annual nacho party, I make a fancy salsa, cashew cream
and guac to go with them.*

1   Preheat the oven to 200°C (400°F/gas 7).

2   Put the corn chips in an ovenproof dish (sheet pan) and top with black beans,
    salsa, cheese and jalapeños or chilli flakes. (I've told Andy that salsa doesn't
    go on until after cooking, but he doesn't believe me. Feel free to put it on
    afterwards if you like. If using homemade salsa, definitely put on afterwards.)

3   Bake in the oven for 10 minutes or until the cheese is melted and bubbling and
    edges of some of the corn chips are starting to turn brown.

4   Remove from the oven and serve on its own, or topped with avocado, cashew
    cream or vegean sour cream and coriander leaves, or any other toppings you
    may wish to add. Devour.

FOR HOMEMADE SALSA:

Combine tinned sweetcorn, finely chopped red onion, tomato, red (bell)
pepper and coriander (cilantro), and heaps of lime juice.

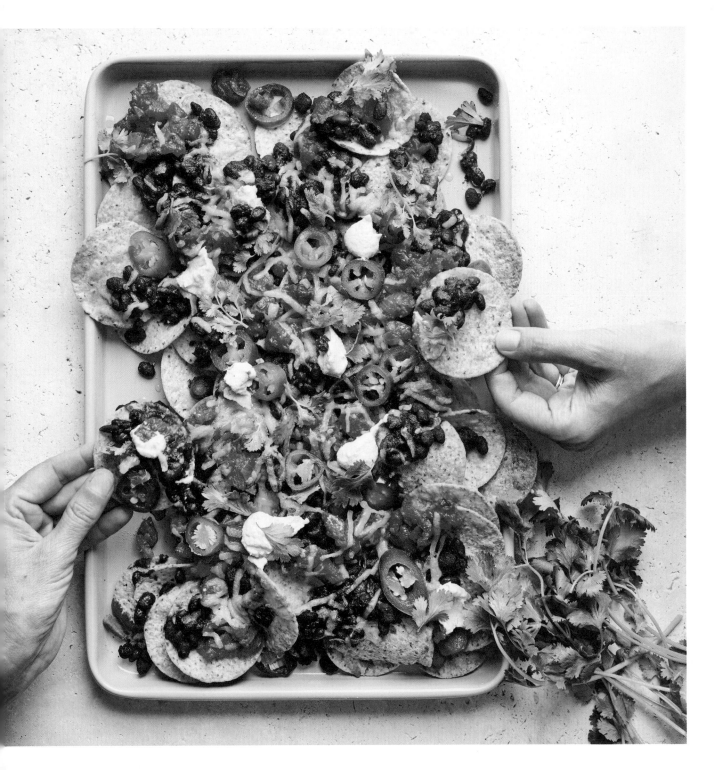

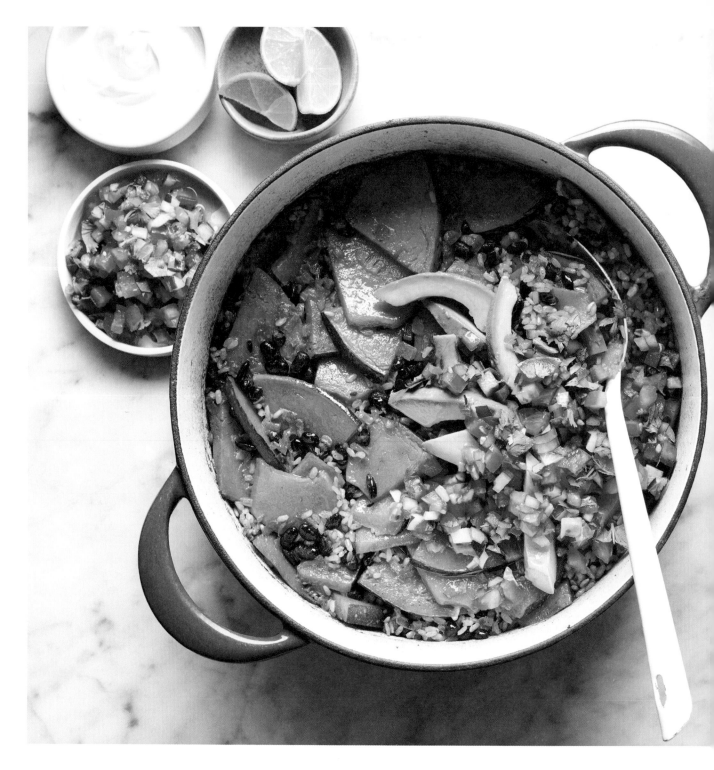

INGREDIENTS

generous glug of olive oil

1 red onion, finely chopped

2 garlic cloves, finely chopped

1½ teaspoons ground cumin

1½ teaspoons ground coriander

1½ teaspoons sweet smoked
paprika

440 g (15½ oz/generous 2 cups)
long-grain white rice

400 g (14 oz) tin black beans,
drained and rinsed (or 260 g/
9½ oz/1½ cups Beloved Black
Beans – page 74 – drained but
not rinsed)

¼ pumpkin or ½ butternut squash
(approx. 500 g/1 lb 2 oz),
halved, seeded and cut into
5 mm- (¼ in-) thick wedges

2 teaspoons salt

1 litre (34 fl oz/4 cups) water

2 tomatoes, finely chopped

1 fresh jalapeño (or ½ green/
(bell) pepper if you can't
do spicy), seeded and finely
chopped

handful of fresh coriander
(cilantro) leaves, finely chopped

To serve:

1 ripe avocado, peeled and diced

1 lime, halved

vegan sour cream or Cashew
Cream (page 22)

Pumpkin and Black Bean Baked Rice

We all need meals in our repertoire that you can prep ahead of time and throw on when you get home, leaving it to cook itself while you take care of any of the bazillion things on your to-do list. This is one of those meals.

1   Preheat the oven to 200°C (400°F/gas 7).

2   Heat the olive oil in a large casserole pot (Dutch oven) or an ovenproof saucepan over a medium-high heat, add three-quarters of the onion, and cook for a couple of minutes until it is starting to go transparent. Add the garlic and spices and cook for a couple of minutes, then add the rice, beans, pumpkin, salt and water. Increase the heat to high then, once the water is simmering, cover with a lid and transfer to the hot oven to cook for 30 minutes.

3   While the pumpkin and rice is cooking, make a simple salsa by combining the reserved finely chopped onion with the chopped tomato, jalapeño and coriander leaves in a small bowl.

4   After 30 minutes, remove the dish from the oven, take off the lid, give it a stir, then serve in bowls and top each serving with the salsa, diced avocado, a squeeze of fresh lime and spoonfuls of sour cream or cashew cream.

5   Leftovers will keep in the refrigerator for up to 4 days, and up to 3 months in the freezer.

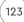

INGREDIENTS
decent glug of olive oil
1 medium red onion,
    finely chopped
2 garlic cloves, finely chopped
1 decent-sized courgette
    (zucchini), halved lengthways
    and cut into thick half-moons
400 g (14 oz) tin butter (lima)
    beans, drained and rinsed
260 g (9½ oz/1 cup) passata
    (sieved tomatoes)
½ teaspoon salt
freshly ground black pepper
dried chilli (hot pepper) flakes
    (optional, but sooo good)
2 sprigs of fresh oregano

To serve:
2 slices of bread, toasted
1–2 tablespoons good-quality
    vegan feta

Baked Butter Beans and Courgette

What this dish lacks in looks it makes up for in flavour. It's the perfect bang together meal that takes care of itself in the oven while I put my kids to bed and is good on those nights where I snack with my kids at dinner time but don't eat a proper dinner and need something to satiate me. It also makes for a delicious breakfast and very easily doubles if you need to stretch it further.

1   Preheat the oven to 220°C (430°F/gas 9).

2   Heat the oil in a large casserole pot (Dutch oven) or an ovenproof saucepan over a medium-high heat, add the onion and cook for 5 minutes until translucent and starting to brown. Add the garlic and stir, then quickly add the courgette and butter beans and stir some more (you don't want the garlic to burn). Add the passata and salt, a pinch of black pepper and some chilli flakes (if using), stir, then cover with a lid and place in the hot oven for 25 minutes. Add the oregano and replace the lid for a moment, while you slice your bread and fetch your feta.

3   Spoon onto the bread and top with feta.

4   Leftovers store well in the refrigerator for up to 4 days and can be reheated in the microwave or on the hob with a splash of water.

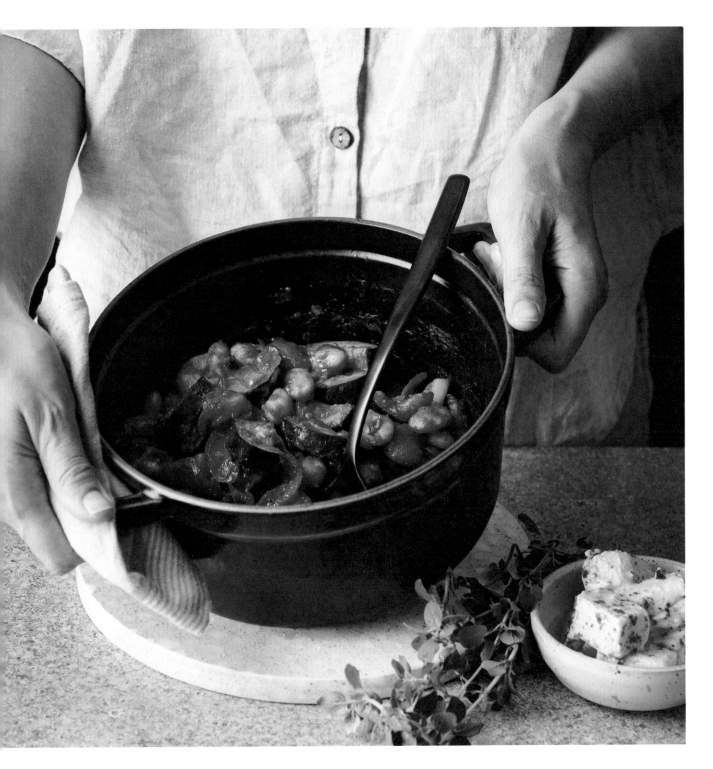

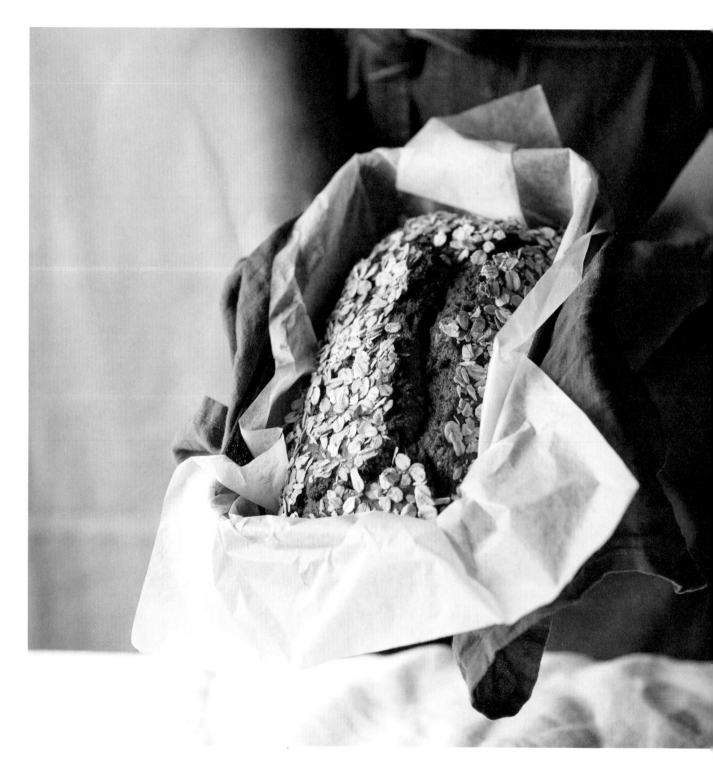

INGREDIENTS

4 bananas, the riper and spottier
   they are, the better
5 tablespoons melted coconut oil
   or olive oil
1 teaspoon bicarbonate of soda
   (baking soda)
180 g (6½ oz/½ cup) rice malt syrup
185 g (6½ oz/1½ cups) plain
   (all-purposed) flour (or see
   Tip for alternatives)
1 teaspoon vanilla extract
pinch of salt

Optional extras:
handful of chopped walnuts,
   pecans or chocolate
a few tablespoons of seeds
spices, such as ground cinnamon
   and nutmeg
good-quality chocolate

For sprinkling:
small handful of chopped nuts,
   seeds, desiccated (shredded)
   or flaked coconut, or oats

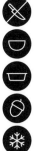

Banana Bread 2.0

This recipe is in my first cookbook but since having children, I have changed the sugar content significantly. It's so simple and versatile and it's a great base for adding all kinds of goodies such as nuts or chocolate. Louie won't eat it if there's walnuts inside, so my current go-to nutrition boost is hemp, chia and flax seeds.

1   Preheat the oven to 180°C (350°F/gas 6) and line a 10 × 25 cm (4 × 10 in) loaf pan with baking paper.

2   Peel the bananas and mash them in a large mixing bowl (not too much – you want the mash a little lumpy). Add the remaining ingredients, one at a time, stirring well after each addition. You want the oil to be fully incorporated before you add the bicarbonate of soda, and the bicarbonate of soda to be fully incorporated before you add the sugar, and the sugar fully incorporated (the batter will look almost white and creamy by now) before you add the flour. Finally, add any nuts or seeds, spices or chocolate, if using, and stir them through.

3   Pour the mixture into the baking paper-lined loaf pan and sprinkle with chopped nuts, seeds, coconut or oats, as I have in this pic.

4   Bake in the hot oven for 45 minutes–1 hour. How long it will take to cook will depend on your loaf pan and oven power, and there's nothing more disappointing than sunken banana bread, so check it by inserting a skewer into the middle of the bread. If it comes out clean, it's ready.

5   Remove the bread from the oven and allow to cool in the pan before devouring.

TIP: I usually only make banana bread with wheat, oat and spelt flours, but I've had success with buckwheat flour and I've had feedback from friends that it's really good with a gluten-free flour blend, too.

MAKES 6–8 SLICES

INGREDIENTS

coconut oil, for greasing
400 ml (14 fl oz) tin coconut milk
   (or any other plant milk)
2 tablespoons chia seeds
1 teaspoon apple cider vinegar
115 g (3¾ oz/⅓ cup) rice malt
   or maple syrup
5 tablespoons olive oil or melted
   coconut oil
225 g (8 oz/2 cups) grated carrot
   (about 3 medium carrots)
200 g (7 oz/2 cups) quick-cook oats
2 teaspoons ground ginger
1 teaspoon ground cinnamon
1 teaspoon vanilla extract
¼ teaspoon ground nutmeg
1 teaspoon bicarbonate of soda
   (baking soda)
1 teaspoon baking powder
pinch of salt
generous handful of walnuts
   (about 60 g/2 oz)
115 g (3¾ oz/¾ cup) fresh or frozen
   blueberries
1–2 tablespoons raw cane sugar
   (optional)

To serve:
coconut yoghurt
finely grated lemon zest (optional)

Carrot and Blueberry Breakfast Cake

This is the perfect marriage of my favourite breakfast food (porridge) and my favourite cake (carrot). Every time I make it I crave it for days on end because hot damn, nothing in the world beats that combination of spices.

So long as you keep the basic ratios the same, there are plenty of substitutions you can make in this recipe – think almond milk instead of soy, sultanas instead of blueberries, etc. It also makes a great toddler snack if you chop the walnuts finely or replace with a safer alternative such as hemp seeds.

1   Preheat the oven to 160°C (320°F/gas 4) and grease the baking pan with coconut oil.

2   Combine the coconut milk, chia seeds and apple cider vinegar in a bowl and allow it to curdle.

3   Add the rice malt or maple syrup, oil and grated carrot to the wet mixture, stir until well combined and then add all the dry ingredients and stir again until well combined. Fold in the blueberries then pour the mixture (apart from the raw cane sugar) into the greased baking pan. Sprinkle with sugar, if using, and place in the hot oven to bake for 30–40 minutes, until golden on top and crisp around the edges.

4   Remove from the oven and allow to sit for 10 minutes before loosening the edges with a metal spatula. Slice in the pan and serve warm, topped with spoonfuls of coconut yoghurt and some lemon zest (if using). Heaven. It can be eaten cold too, but I prefer it warm as the spices are more prominent and the contrast of hot cake with cold and melty yoghurt is really incredible.

5   Store leftovers in the refrigerator for up to 4 days and enjoy hot or at room temperature, but always with yoghurt. It also freezes well.

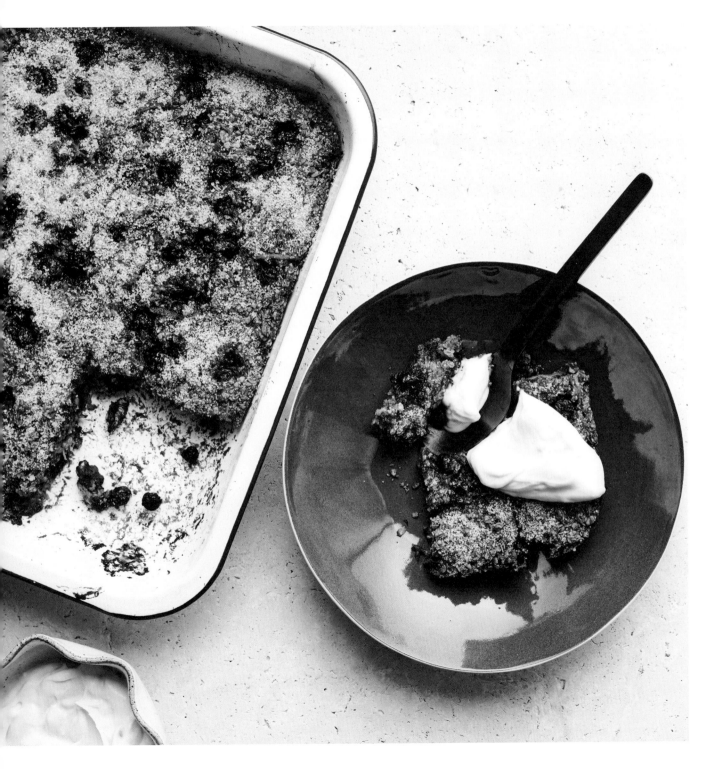

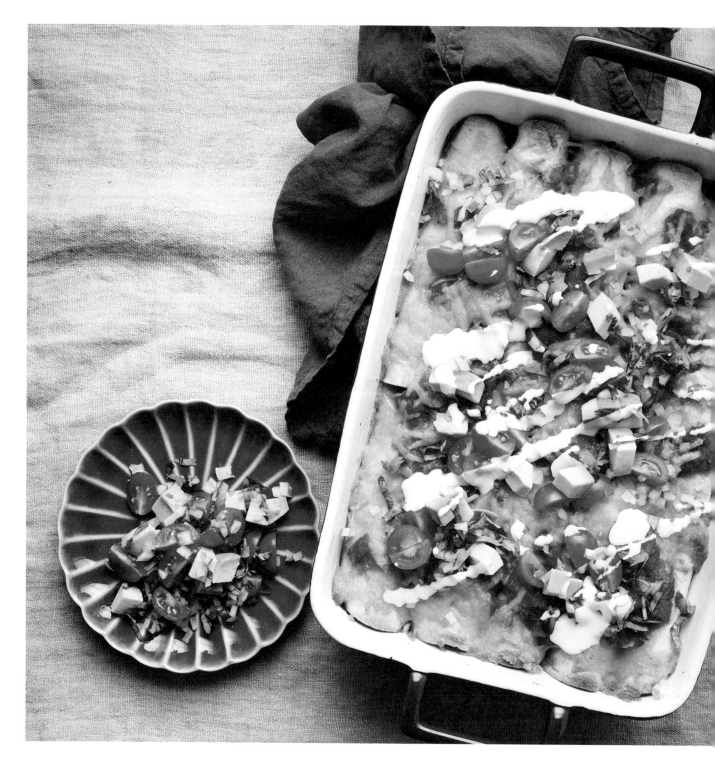

SERVES 4

INGREDIENTS

2 × 400 g (14 oz) tins black beans,
    drained and rinsed (or 500 g/
    1 lb 2 oz/3 cups Beloved Black Beans
    (page 74) drained but not rinsed)
400 g (14 oz) tin sweetcorn, drained
1 heaped teaspoon salt
1 heaped teaspoon onion powder
1 heaped teaspoon garlic powder
1 heaped teaspoon ground coriander
1 heaped teaspoon ground cumin
1 heaped teaspoon sweet smoked
    paprika
about 100 g (3½ oz) vegan cream
    cheese or Cashew Cream (page 22),
    vegan sour cream, etc., plus extra for
    topping
10–12 wheat tortillas (about 12 cm/4½ in)
450 g (1 lb) jar chunky Mexican
    tomato salsa
100 g (3½ oz) good-quality vegan
    hard cheese, grated
small handful of fresh coriander
    (cilantro), finely chopped (optional)

For the topping (optional):
1 ripe avocado
1 tomato
¼ fresh or pickled red onion
handful of fresh coriander
    (cilantro) leaves
handful of fresh sliced or pickled
    jalapeño

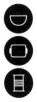

Easiest Enchiladas

This recipe takes some long life pantry items, freshens them up with a bit of a chunky salsa on top and boom! A gourmet midweek meal that makes a perfect leftover meal for breakfast, lunch or dinner the following day.

1   Preheat the oven to 200°C (400°F/gas 7).

2   Combine the beans, sweetcorn, salt and spices in a large mixing bowl. Add your cream cheese or cashew cream and use a potato masher to combine everything.

3   Get your tortillas and figure out the best way to pack them into your baking dish so you have a rough idea where to place them before you begin. I do two rows of 6, but your configuration will depend on the size of your tortillas and dish. Don't be fussy; you can squish them in and it will be crazy delicious. Pour half the jar of salsa into the bottom of the baking dish. Place a heaped tablespoon of bean and corn filling into a tortilla, roll it up and place it seam side down in the sauce. Repeat with all the tortillas then cover with the remaining salsa and the grated cheese.

4   Place in the hot oven and bake for 20 minutes. While they are cooking, prepare your toppings, if using, cutting everything as small as you can be bothered. I find it easier to get a good amount per enchilada when the toppings are finely chopped. If using cream cheese, thin it out with some water to get it to a pourable consistency. If using cashew cream or vegan sour cream, skip this step.

5   Once cooked, remove the enchiladas from oven, sprinkle with toppings (if using), pour over the creamy element, then serve.

> TIP: For extra smoky heat, use chipotle sauce in the bean mix or on top of the enchiladas.

INGREDIENTS
generous glug of olive oil
1 red onion, diced
1 teaspoon ground cumin
1 teaspoon ground coriander
1 roasted red (bell) pepper
    (from a jar), finely chopped
2–3 garlic cloves, finely chopped
stalks from a bunch of fresh
    coriander (cilantro), finely
    chopped (save the leaves
    for garnishing)
2 × 400 g (14 oz) tins chopped
    tomatoes
2 × 400 g (14 oz) tins black beans,
    drained but not rinsed
1 teaspoon salt
1 tablespoon sugar
freshly cracked black pepper

To serve:
1 ripe avocado, peeled and diced
4–8 tablespoons Cashew Cream
    (page 22) or something else
    creamy
pickled jalapeños or any other
    spicy ingredient of your choice
    in fresh, dried or sauce form

Baked Black Beans

This dish has so much flavour, and is a great way to use tinned black beans. At the risk of sounding like a broken record, you can serve in a million different ways, whether on its own, on toast, over a baked potato, with corn chips, wrapped in burritos with some salady fillings, etc.

You can also turn it into a brunch feast by serving with really good potatoes, scrambled tofu, cashew cream and guac, and either corn chips or soft shell tacos.

1   Preheat the oven to 220°C (430°F/gas 9).

2   Heat the olive oil in a large casserole pot (Dutch oven) or an ovenproof saucepan over a medium-high heat, add the onion and cook for about 5 minutes until soft and starting to brown. Add the cumin, coriander, red pepper, garlic and coriander stalks and cook for a few minutes, until softened and well combined. Add the tomatoes, beans, salt and sugar, season with black pepper and give it a good stir. Cover with a lid and place in the hot oven for 30 minutes, removing the lid for the final 5 minutes of cooking.

3   Remove from the oven and serve on its own, or with one of the accompaniments listed in the intro, topped with diced avocado, cashew cream, jalapeños or other chilli, and reserved coriander leaves, or any other toppings you may wish to add.

4   Leftovers will keep in the refrigerator for up to 4 days.

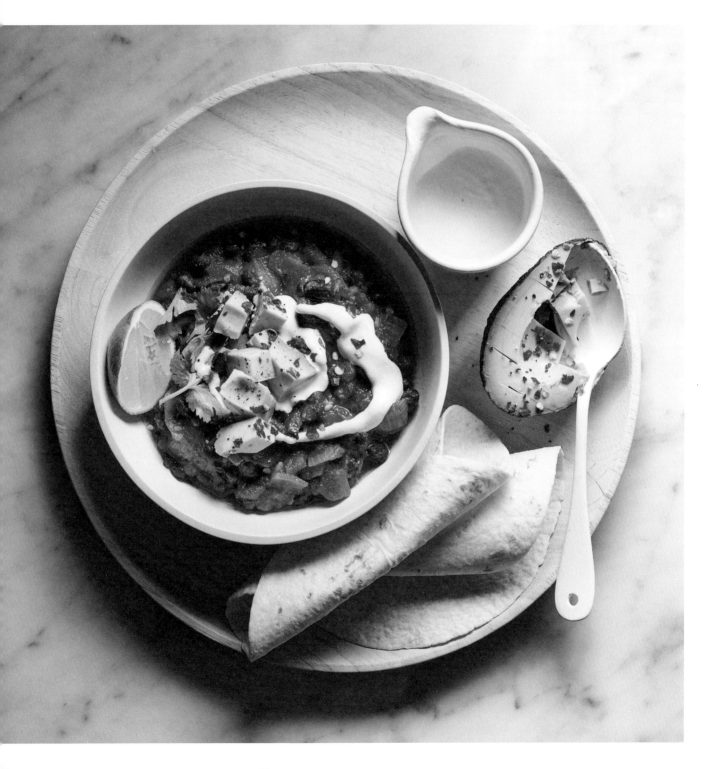

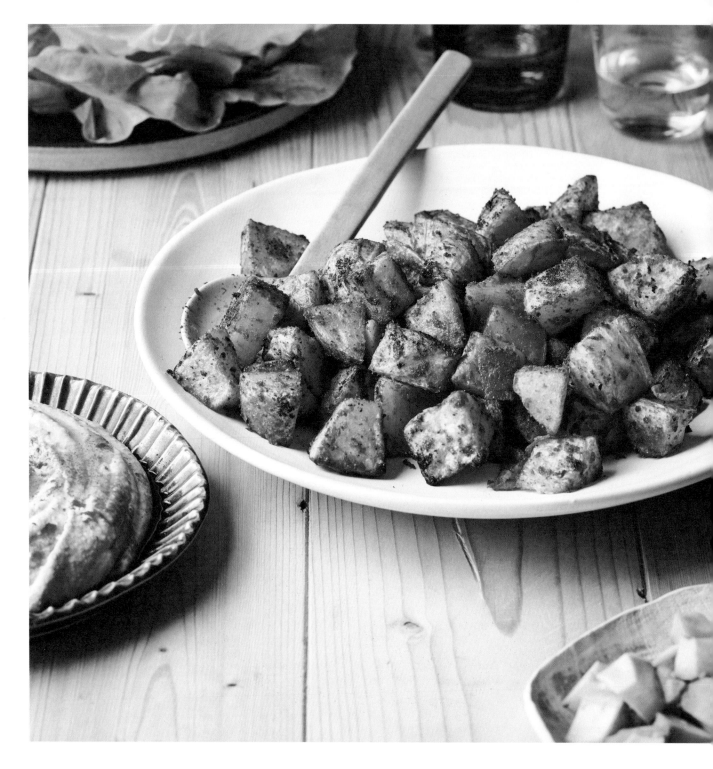

INGREDIENTS
1.2 kg (2 lb 6 oz) potatoes, peeled
    and cut into 1 cm (½ in) cubes
generous glug of olive oil
3 tablespoons Really
    Good Potato Seasoning
    (page 27)

To serve (optional):
hummus (store-bought or
    homemade – see recipe
    on page 21)
1 ripe avocado, peeled and diced
a couple of heads of lettuce,
    leaves separated to make cups

Really Good Potatoes

These potatoes are a real crowd pleaser – every time I make them, someone asks for the recipe. The combination of spices is so good and I highly recommend having a jar of it made up at all times so you can whip up these as a dinner or side with very little effort.

I always go for kipfler or Dutch cream potatoes if buying specifically for this dish, but waxy potatoes roast beautifully too. You can also make this recipe with sweet potatoes, which I do often.

1 Preheat the oven to 220°C (430°F/gas 9).

2 Toss the potatoes in the oil and seasoning mix then spread them over one or two oven trays (sheet pans) (two if you can, as the more room they have, the crispier they will get, but one is totally fine too).

3 Roast the potatoes in the oven for 20 minutes or until golden brown, with slightly darker edges. You should be able to easily pierce them with a fork.

4 Enjoy immediately, as they are, or with hummus, diced avocado and lettuce cups, or with any number of dishes in this book.

SERVES 4-8

INGREDIENTS
generous glug of olive oil
1 onion, diced
300 g (10½ oz) vegan sausages,
    cut into 1 cm (½ in)-thick slices
about 300 g (10½ oz) stale bread,
    ripped into bite-size pieces
4 large Tuscan kale leaves,
    tough stems removed
    and leaves chopped
 2 garlic cloves, finely chopped
750 ml (25 fl oz/3 cups) vegan
    'beef' stock

Sausage and Kale Bready Bake

Reminiscent of an American style 'stuffing', this dish is comfort food at its finest. It's loved by vegans and omnivores alike, making it the perfect thing to take to a Christmas or Thanksgiving feast.

1   Preheat the oven to 200°C (400°F/gas 7).

2   Heat a glug of the oil in an ovenproof frying pan (skillet) over a medium heat, add the onion and cook for a few minutes, until it starts to brown. Add the sausages and cook for 5–10 minutes until crispy and golden brown all over. Transfer the onions and sausages to a plate.

3   Add a drizzle more oil to the pan, add the bread and cook, stirring often, for 5–10 minutes until it starts to brown. Add the kale and cook for about 5 minutes until soft. Put the onion and sausages back into the pan, along with the garlic and stock. Nestle the kale leaves under the stock to prevent them from burning, then place in the hot oven and bake for 30 minutes until the top is golden and the stock has been absorbed by the bread. Remove from the oven and serve.

4   The 'stuffing' is best eaten hot, but also really good at room temperature, and we know how important room-temp foods are for Christmas. It will also keep for up to 4 days in the refrigerator.

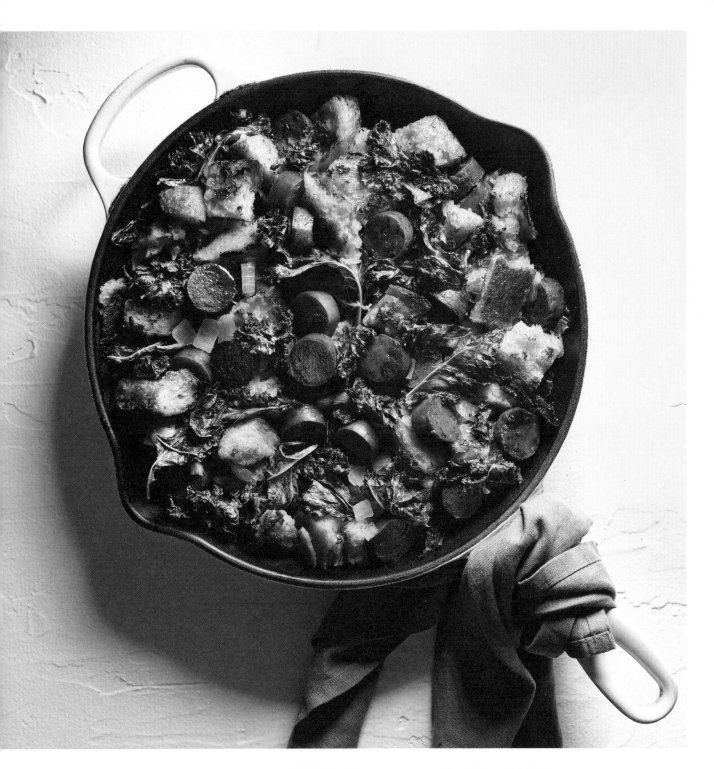

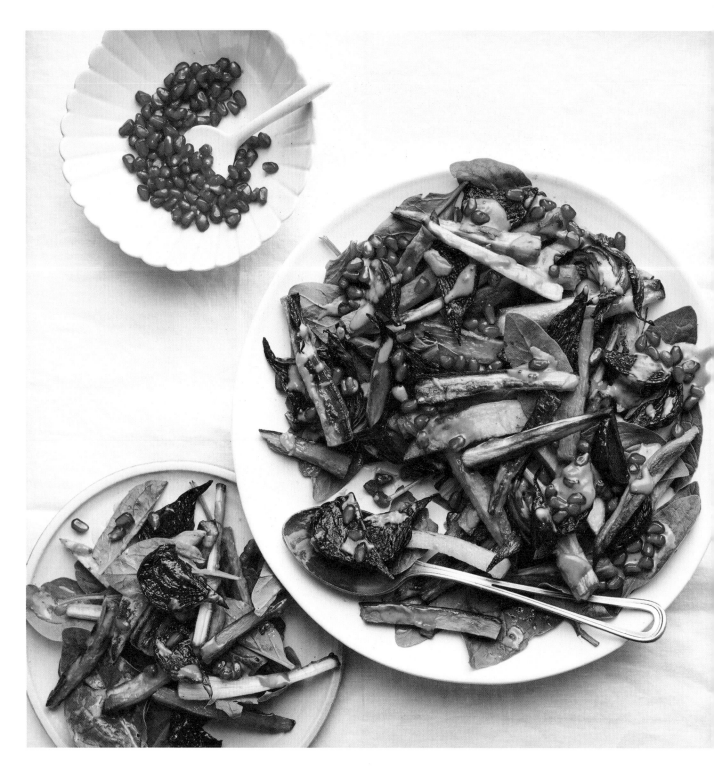

INGREDIENTS

For the roast veg:

about 200–300 g (7–10½ oz)
of:
- 2 parsnips
- 2 carrots
- 2 potatoes
- 2 sweet potatoes
- 2 beetroots (beets)

peeled and chopped into
cubes or wedges about
1–2.5 cm (½–1 in) in size
1 red onion, cut into wedges
(root kept intact)
1 bulb of garlic, cut in half
olive oil, for drizzling (or
an olive oil spray)
generous sprinkle of sea salt
handful of chopped walnuts

For the rest of the salad:

3–4 handfuls of baby spinach
seeds from ½ pomegranate

For the dressing:

3 tablespoons olive oil
2 tablespoons balsamic vinegar
1 tablespoon maple syrup
1 teaspoon wholegrain mustard
1 teaspoon salt
100 g (3½ oz) tahini
3–5 tablespoons cold water, to thin
freshly ground black pepper

Roasted Root Vegetable Salad with Tahini and Pomegranate

Another nostalgic one, this salad reminds me of my first Christmas in Berlin in 2012. Roasted vegetable salads are my jam – I've been making them my entire life – but the combination of tahini dressing and pomegranate seeds was a new discovery for me that I am addicted to forever more.

1   Preheat the oven to 200°C (400°F/gas 7).

2   Arrange the vegetable wedges, onion and garlic on a large roasting tray (over two trays if necessary) and coat them with olive oil and the salt. (I like to use my olive oil spray here, to ensure an even coating.) Place in the hot oven to roast for 40–50 minutes, tossing the vegetables once during the cooking time and adding the walnuts for the final 10 minutes of cooking. Once the veggies are golden in colour and can be easily pierced with the tip of a knife, remove from the oven and allow to cool for 10 minutes.

3   While the veggies are cooking, combine all the dressing ingredients, except the water, in a jar or small bowl and set aside.

4   Once the veggies are cooked and the garlic is cool enough to touch, squeeze the cooked garlic from the papery skins and add it to the dressing. Stir really well and add enough water to thin the dressing to a loose, pourable consistency.

5   Add the baby spinach to the veggies on the tray and toss to combine. Drizzle the entire salad with the dressing, toss once more and then scatter pomegranate seeds over it. Serve immediately, on the tray(s) you cooked the veggies on.

6   If not eating immediately, wait until the veggies are cool before tossing with spinach (or it will wilt) and save the dressing and pomegranate seeds for just before serving. The veggies will keep in the refrigerator for up to 4 days.

SERVES 4–6

INGREDIENTS

For the dressing:

120 ml (4 fl oz/½ cup) olive oil

60 ml (2 fl oz/¼ cup) apple cider vinegar

2 tablespoons maple syrup

2 teaspoons wholegrain mustard

1 garlic clove, finely chopped

For the salad:

1 whole cauliflower, cut into bite-size florets, stalk trimmed and cut into bite-size pieces

olive oil

1 teaspoon salt

1 teaspoon ground cumin

400 g (14 oz) tin lentils (green or brown), drained and rinsed

a few handfuls of baby spinach or rocket (arugula)

handful of currants

handful of capers (baby capers)

handful of toasted flaked (sliced) almonds

handful of chopped pistachios

fresh coriander (cilantro), to taste

Roasted Cauliflower Salad

At the time of writing this book, this was my go-to salad for so many meals with friends. You can prep it ahead of time if you are having people over for a feast, and it travels really well if you are going to somewhere and wish to take something with you.

Cauliflower is my favourite veggie to use in this salad but you can experiment with other veggies and different nuts, e.g. pumpkin and pine nuts or sweet potato and walnuts, just keep the basic ratios the same and you are guaranteed to have a killer salad.

1   Preheat the oven to 190°C (375°F/gas 6).

2   Make the dressing by putting all the ingredients in a screw top lidded jar, screwing on the lid and giving it a good shake. Set aside.

3   Coat the cauliflower in the oil, salt and cumin, either in a bowl or directly on a baking tray (sheet). Spread the cauliflower evenly across the baking tray and place in the hot oven for 20 minutes, or until edges of the florets are slightly blackened. (If your almonds aren't already toasted, add them for the final 3 minutes of cooking time.)

4   When cooked, remove from the oven and allow to cool for 10 minutes then add the lentils, spinach or rocket, currants, capers, toasted almonds, chopped pistachios and fresh coriander. Drizzle with the dressing, toss and devour.

5   Leftovers will keep in the refrigerator for up to 3 days. Serve cold.

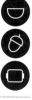

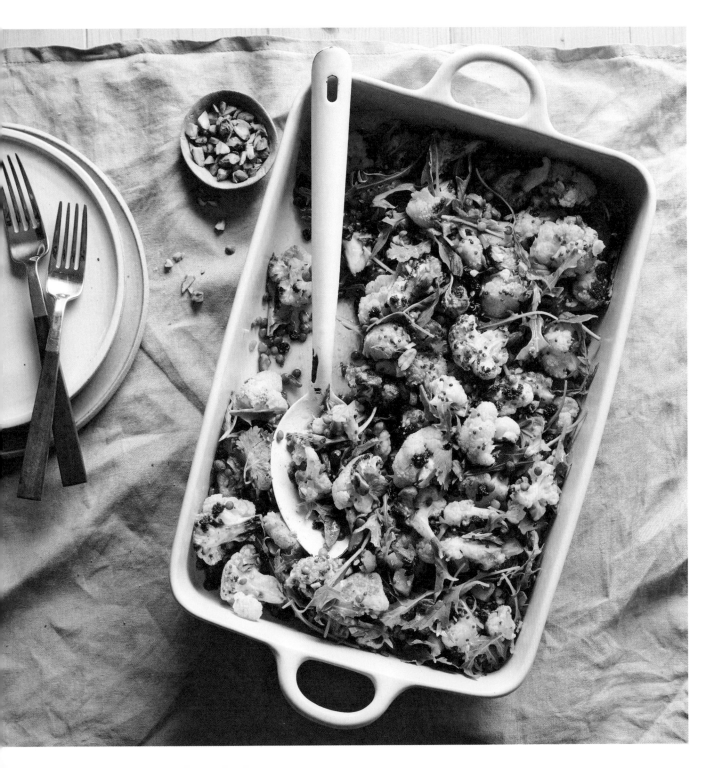

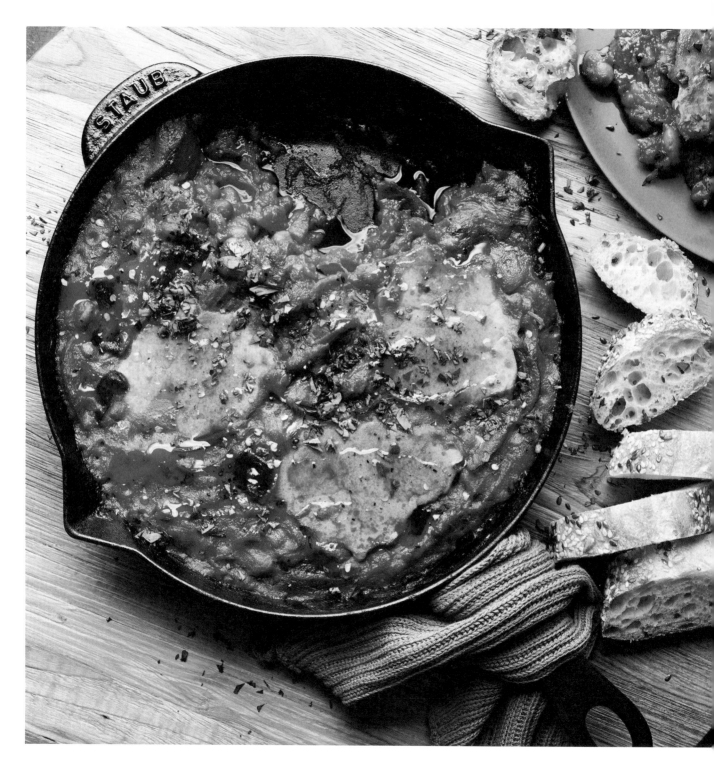

SERVES 2–4

INGREDIENTS

For the 'eggs':

140 g (4½ oz/1¼ cups) chickpea
  (gram) flour
120 ml (4 fl oz/½ cup) warm water
60 ml (2 fl oz/¼ cup) olive oil
¾ teaspoon black salt
¾ teaspoon onion powder
¾ teaspoon garlic powder

For the sauce:

generous glug of olive oil
1 red onion, diced
1 teaspoon ground cumin
1 roasted red (bell) pepper
  (from a jar), finely chopped
2–3 garlic cloves, finely chopped
2 × 400 g (14 oz) tins chopped
  tomatoes
400 g (14 oz) tin borlotti
  (cranberry) beans, drained
  and rinsed
1 teaspoon salt
1 tablespoon sugar
freshly cracked black pepper

To serve:

finely chopped fresh parsley
toasted bread or pita

Something Like Shakshuka

Shakshuka is a Middle Eastern dish of eggs cooked in tomato sauce, that can be served in a kazillion different ways depending on where you are eating it and who's cooking it.

Borlotti beans are not at all a Middle Eastern bean but I find that they meld into the sauce really beautifully, becoming a part of it rather than standing out as a thing that's there for the sauce. You can swap them for pinto beans, cannellini (white) beans or chickpeas (garbanzos) if you prefer.

1 Preheat the oven to 200°C (400°F/gas 7).

2 Combine all the 'egg' ingredients in a bowl and whisk until smooth. Set aside for 30 minutes.

3 Heat the olive oil in an ovenproof frying pan (skillet) or saucepan (that has a lid) over a medium-high heat, add the diced onion and cook for about 5 minutes until soft and starting to brown. Add the cumin, red pepper and garlic and cook for a couple of minutes, then add the tomatoes, beans, salt, sugar and a generous pinch of black pepper and give it a good stir. Once it's bubbling, make a little well in the tomato mixture and add chickpea flour 'eggs' into the sauce by placing 2 heaped tablespoons of batter into the well, one on top of the other. Do this in 4 different wells in the pan. Don't worry if they aren't perfect circles.

4 Cover with a lid and place in the hot oven for 20 minutes. Remove from the oven and sprinkle with parsley. Serve with toasted bread or stuffed inside a fluffy and delicious pita.

INGREDIENTS

160 g (5½ oz/generous ½ cup)
    maple syrup
200 g (7 oz/generous ¾ cup)
    smooth and runny peanut
    butter
90 g (3¼ oz/scant 1 cup)
    ground almonds
90 g (3¼ oz/scant 1 cup)
    quick-cook oats
1½ teaspoons baking powder
30 g (1 oz/¼ cup) cocoa powder
40 g (1½ oz/¼ cup) hemp seeds
1 teaspoon vanilla extract
pinch of salt

The World's Healthiest Chocolate Cookies

My sister-in-law is obsessed with these cookies. The perfect thing to whip up when you have impromptu visitors and no snacks in the house, they are low mess, come together in moments and cook just as quickly. They are also the perfect thing to whip up in early labour while trying to kill time, or for a friend who has just had a baby.

I weigh everything direct into the bowl so that I don't have any measuring cups, etc., to wash at the end of cooking.

1   Preheat the oven to 180°C (350°F/gas 6) and line a baking tray (sheet pan) with baking paper.

2   Combine the maple syrup and peanut butter (heated gently if necessary, to loosen) in a bowl. Add the dry ingredients and mix to combine.

3   Roll the mixture into 15 balls and place the balls on the lined baking tray. Flatten them until they are about 1 cm (½ in) thick and bake in the hot oven for 8–10 minutes, or until you can smell them.

4   Remove from the oven and allow to cool on the tray.

5   The cookies will keep in an airtight jar for up to 1 month.

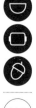

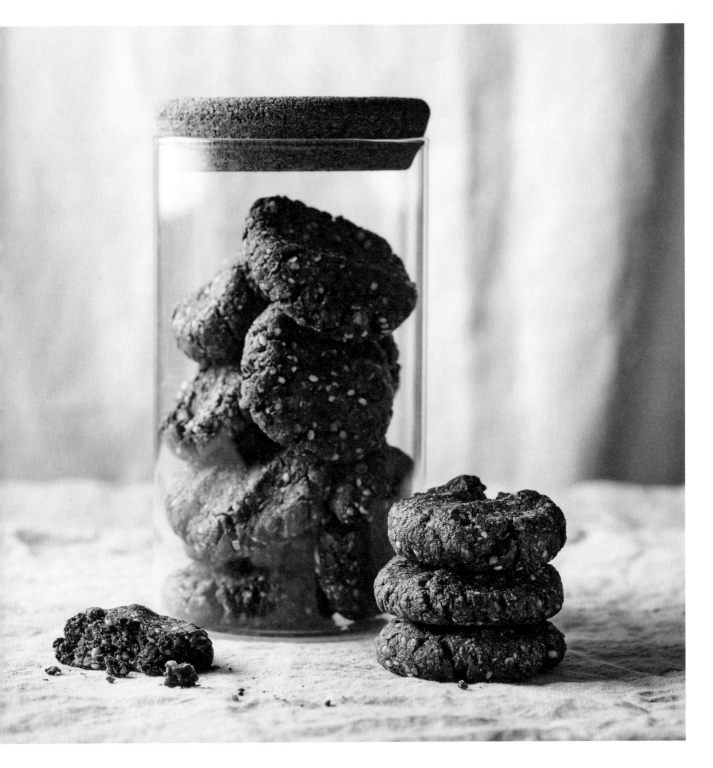

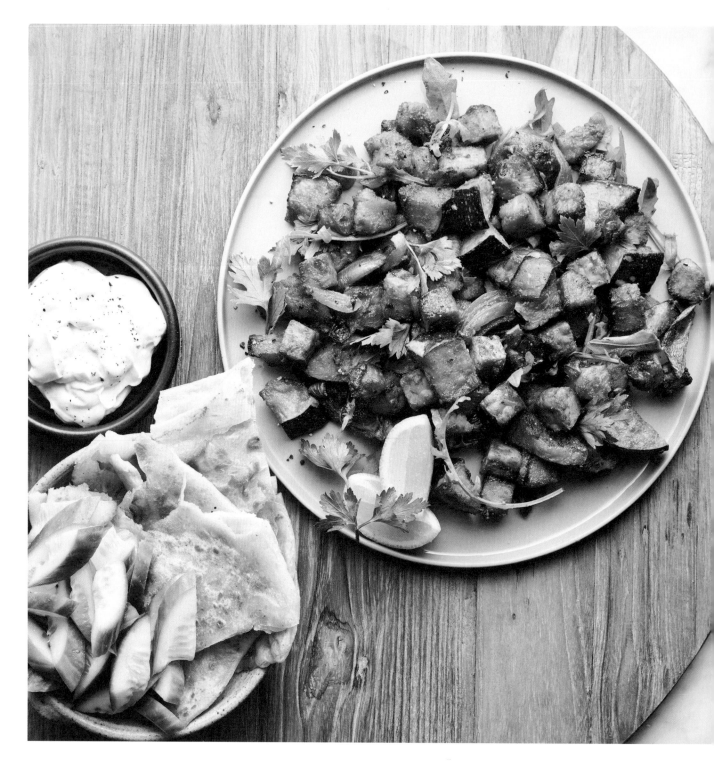

INGREDIENTS

60 ml (2 fl oz/¼ cup) melted
     coconut oil
60 ml (2 fl oz/¼ cup) maple syrup
1 tablespoon curry powder
1 teaspoon salt
about 500 g (1 lb 2 oz) pumpkin
     or butternut squash, seeded
     and cut into bite-size pieces
     (skin on, unless tough)
about 225 g (8 oz) tempeh,
     cut into 1 cm (½ in) cubes
1 red onion, cut into wedges
     (root kept intact)
2–3 handfuls of rocket (arugula)
     or baby spinach
1 small cucumber, diced
handful of fresh coriander
     (cilantro) leaves, finely chopped

To serve:

1 lemon, halved
250 g (9 oz/1 cup) coconut
     yoghurt
2–4 restaurant-bought garlic
     naan or roti (optional, but
     soooo good)

Sweet, Sticky Curried Tempeh Tray Bake

Tempeh is an excellent source of protein, yet many people are baffled as to how to prepare it. It has a bitterness, which can be removed with steaming; however, I prefer to marinate the bejeesus out of it and hide the bitterness with sweetness and spices. This tray bake is a winner for a quick weeknight meal, or to prep ahead of time for lunches during the week.

1   Preheat the oven to 200°C (400°F/gas 7).

2   Combine the coconut oil, maple syrup, curry powder and salt in a small bowl and set aside.

3   Place the pumpkin, tempeh and onion in a high-edged baking tray (pan). Pour the curry powder concoction over it and use your hands to evenly coat everything in the marinade, resisting the urge to separate the onion layers from one another as they will do this on their own when you toss them. Wash your hands and transfer the baking tray to the hot oven. Bake for 45 minutes, using a spatula to give everything a good toss and stir about halfway through cooking.

4   Check that the pumpkin can be easily pierced with the tip of a knife and the edges are starting to blacken, then remove the baking tray from the oven and allow to cool for 5 minutes. Loosen everything with a spatula then top with rocket or spinach, cucumber and coriander.

5   To serve, squeeze lemon juice over the top, then dollop coconut yoghurt over everything and lightly toss. Enjoy immediately, either as it is, or using naan (garlic, always) that you've picked up from your local Indian restaurant on your way home to make little mouthfuls with one of each ingredient, and to mop up the juices left in the pan. It's. SO. Good.

INGREDIENTS

For the socca:

140 g (4½ oz/1¼ cup) chickpea
flour (gram flour)

250 ml (8½ fl oz/1 cup) warm water

60 ml (2 fl oz/¼ cup) olive oil,
plus extra for greasing

½ teaspoon salt

Optional extras:

1 red onion, cut into rings

leaves from 1–2 sprigs
of fresh rosemary

Toppings:

pesto or hummus
(page 21 for my pesto
and hummus recipes)

leftover roast veggies

frozen peas, defrosted
(I just let them defrost in
a bowl on the work surface)

rocket (arugula)

fresh herbs

micro-greens

vegan feta

Socca

Socca is a staple in our home. It's a chickpea flour (gram flour) pancake, which is delicious served on its own but also a good way to use up fridge leftovers such as hummus, pesto, sauces, cooked veggies, leafy greens, etc. If you wish to turn it into something more substantial.

The batter needs at least 30 minutes to rest but you can make it in the morning and pop it in the fridge, ready to be cooked when you get home. My kids love this, so if I am feeding it to them too, I double the mixture, make theirs first and let it cool while I make the second one.

1   Combine all the socca ingredients in a bowl or jug and whisk until smooth. Leave to sit for at least 30 minutes.

2   About 30 minutes before you are ready to eat, place a cast-iron ovenproof frying pan (skillet) in your oven so it's right under the grill (broiler) and turn your oven on high (just bake mode, not grill mode for now). Once the oven is hot, carefully remove the frying pan and cover the base with a generous amount of oil. Pour the batter into the hot pan and add the onion rings and/or rosemary if using. Carefully return it to the oven, close the oven door and flick the setting/function to grill, still leaving it on the highest temperature setting.

3   Cook the socca for 10 minutes and then check it: it should be blistered and golden brown on the top, like in the photo.

4   Use a metal spatula to transfer it from the frying pan to a wooden board. Add toppings if you are doing so, then cut into 6 slices.

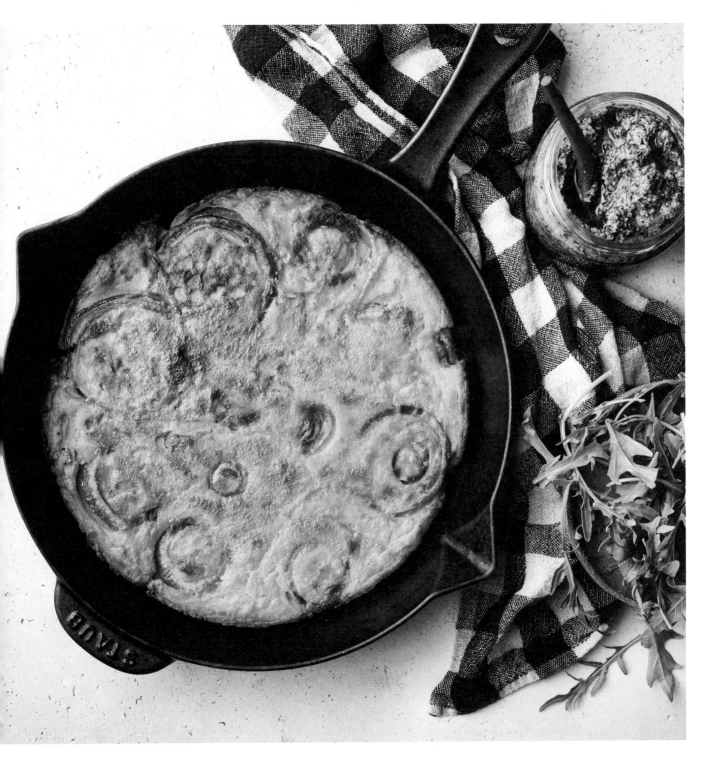

INGREDIENTS

For the roasted chickpeas:

2 × 400 g (14 oz) tins chickpeas
(garbanzos), drained and rinsed
60 ml (2 fl oz/¼ cup) olive oil
1 teaspoon ground coriander
1 teaspoon ground cumin
1 teaspoon sweet smoked paprika
1 teaspoon onion powder
1 teaspoon garlic powder
1 teaspoon salt
1 tablespoon nutritional yeast
2 Lebanese flatbreads, torn into
bite-size pieces
handful of flaked (sliced) almonds
olive oil spray (optional)

For the rest of the salad:

2–3 handfuls of greens such as rocket
(arugula), spinach or baby kale
1 cucumber, sliced into 2 mm-thick rounds
1 ripe avocado, peeled and diced
large handful of fresh mint leaves,
finely chopped
large handful of fresh parsley leaves,
finely chopped

For the dressing:

125 g (4 oz/½ cup) coconut yoghurt
140 g (4½ oz/½ cup) tahini
60 ml (2 fl oz/¼ cup) water
1 teaspoon salt
1 teaspoon maple syrup
juice of 1 lemon
2–3 garlic cloves, crushed (minced)

Warm Chickpea Salad

Always a crowd pleaser, this salad is inspired by fatteh – one of my favourite Middle Eastern dishes.

1   Preheat the oven to 200°C (400°F/gas 7).

2   Put the chickpeas in a deep baking tray (pan) and pat them dry with a clean tea towel. Drizzle with the olive oil then sprinkle with the spices, onion powder, garlic powder and salt and use a spoon to stir and get all the chickpeas nicely covered in oily, spicy goodness. Place in the hot oven and roast for 30 minutes, giving the chickpeas a stir about halfway through cooking.

3   While the chickpeas are in the oven, make the dressing. Place all the ingredients in a small bowl or screw-top jar and stir or shake until well combined. Add more water if you need to, to get it to a pourable consistency. Taste and adjust the salt and maple syrup if necessary, then set aside.

4   Add the flatbread and almonds to the baking dish (spraying the flatbread with oil if you like), and return to the oven for another 5 minutes, or until the bread is lightly golden and crispy.

5   Remove the chickpeas and flatbread from the oven and allow to sit for a few minutes then loosen from the bottom of the dish using a spatula.

6   Just before you are ready to eat, top the chickpeas and flatbread with leafy greens, cucumber slices, diced avocado, mint and parsley. Enjoy immediately, with a generous drizzle of dressing. Leftovers will keep in the refrigerator for up to 4 days.

> TIPS: If you have pita crisps, you can make this salad without turning on the oven! Cook the chickpeas in a frying pan (skillet) instead, for 5–10 minutes until crispy and golden, then add the spices, onion powder, garlic powder and salt and cook for another couple of minutes.
>
> Swap the nutritional yeast and spices for 3 tablespoons of the Really Good Potato Seasoning (page 27) if you like.

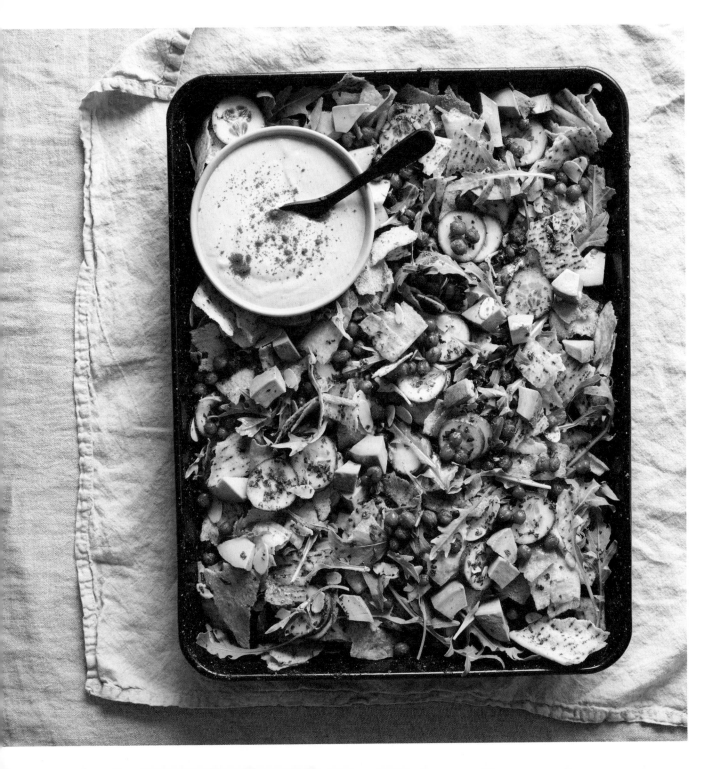

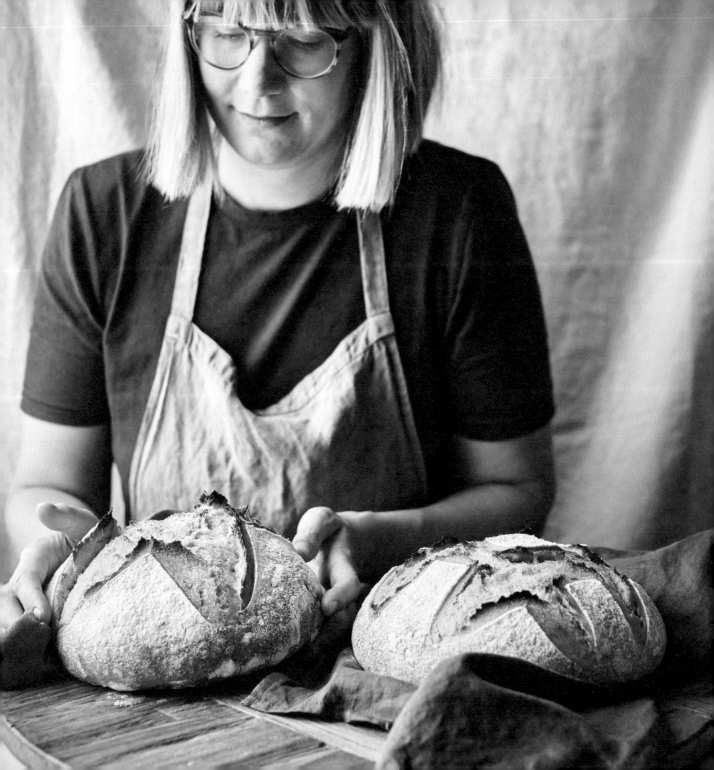

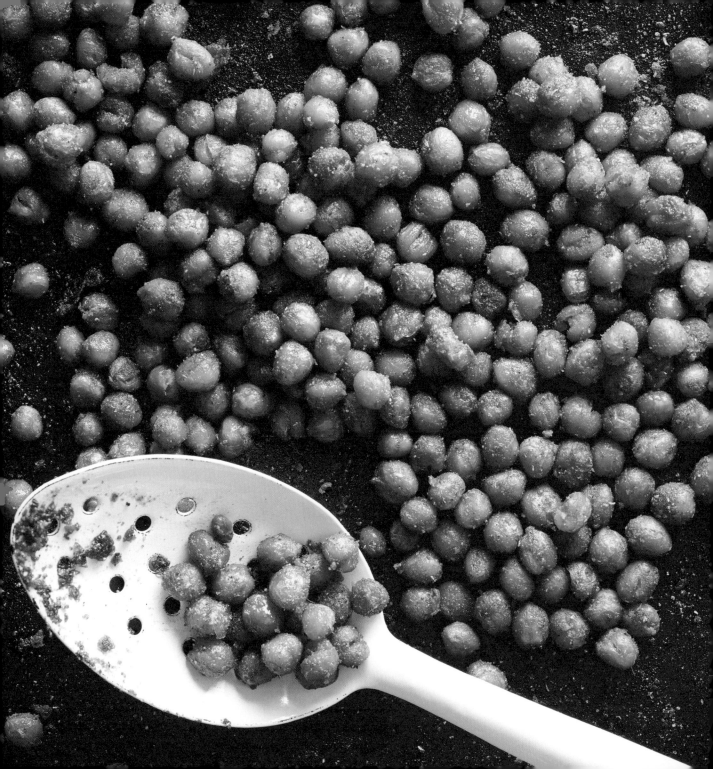

Thanks

Jude. This book is dedicated to you but it is also here because of you. Your demands to be in my arms at all times during the first 10 months of your life is what pushed me to write a book filled with quick, easy, delicious, versatile and low-mess recipes. Your demands to taste every single thing I put in my mouth, and then to taste more and more again, fills me with more joy than you will ever know.

Louie. It all started with you in my belly!! Three books in and here we are, you still don't really like my cooking or understand what I do for a job but you take it all in your stride like the little champ that you are. Thank you for being so patient with me when I am in the kitchen and writing down recipe notes. I love you more than you will ever know.

Andy. My MVP, always. Thank you for putting up with all of my weird food experiments and for being such a great dad to our kids so I can do my job. Writing a book is kind of like having a baby – the final stretch is so hard, so all encompassing, and every time you are in the thick of it you want to throw your hands up in despair and quit. And then it's all over, you forget how hard it was and you want to do it all over again. You've been by my side with great playlists and kind words of encouragement through two babies and three books now. We both know there is no end in sight and I cannot think of a better person to share this journey with.

Mum, Kev, Mand and Steve, for your endless support and encouragement.

My friends and family. Especially Gemma, but everyone else who has eaten my food, tested my recipes, loaned me props for shoots, given me words of encouragement and shared your own delicious creations with me; you inspire me endlessly.

Kajal, Eila and the rest of the folks at Hardie Grant UK for having continual faith in me and letting the creation and shooting of this book unfold across the oceans.

Claire, your ability to take my words and lay them out into something so beautiful and easy to understand, it's quite literally witchcraft. You understand my brain even better than I do, and I am eternally grateful for your design expertise. And Rich, your illustrations have once again captured everything I wanted them to and I am so lucky to have your work between these pages.

My Dream Team! Emma, Deb and Bec who worked tirelessly to cook, style and shoot this book and bring my recipes to life. There was a lot of surrender in having a team involved after flying solo for my previous books, but doing so with you by my side felt so right and I learnt an enormous amount from you all.

Lauren and Jane, for your scrupulous proofreading eye.

Sophie Jane Moran, for the generous loan of your beautiful ceramics.

And last but definitely not least, you, dear reader! Thank you for supporting me so I can continue doing what I love.

About Jessica

Jessica Prescott really likes cooking. She grew up in New Zealand and after many years of living abroad, now resides in Melbourne, Australia with her husband Andy and their two sons, Louie and Jude. This book is her third in a series of vegan cookbooks which share recipes and ideas that are easy and delicious whilst being kind to the planet. When she's not juggling motherhood and recipe writing, you can find Jess in the kitchen of Mama Goodness, creating wholesome and nutritious meals for new mothers.

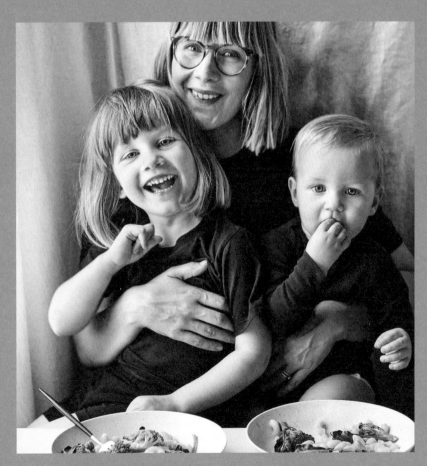

Index

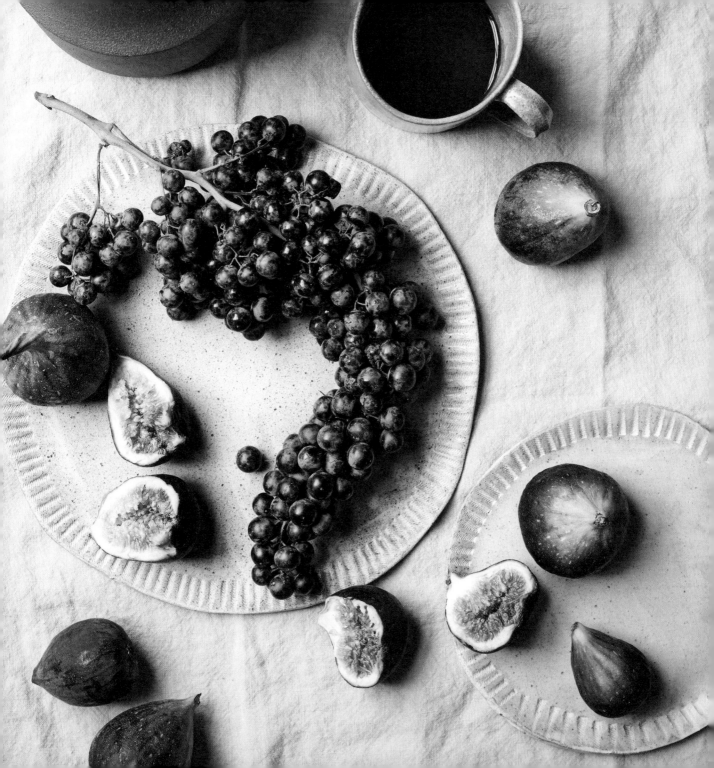

Published in 2020 by Hardie Grant
Books, an imprint of Hardie Grant
Publishing

Hardie Grant Books (London)
5th & 6th Floors
52–54 Southwark Street
London SE1 1UN

Hardie Grant Books (Melbourne)
Building 1, 658 Church Street
Richmond, Victoria 3121

hardiegrantbooks.com

British Library Cataloguing-in-
Publication Data. A catalogue record
for this book is available from the
British Library.

Vegan One-Pot Wonders
ISBN: 978–1–78488–323–2

10 9 8 7 6 5 4 3 2 1

Publishing Director: Kate Pollard
Commissioning Editor: Kajal Mistry
Design: Claire Warner Studio
Illustrator: Richard Robinson
Photographer: Bec Hudson Photography
Food and Prop Stylist: Deborah Kaloper
Home Economist: Emma Rooke
Copy-editor: Laura Nickoll
Editor: Eila Purvis
Proofreader: Jane Bamforth
Indexer: Cathy Heath

Colour reproduction by p2d
Printed and bound in China by
Leo Paper Products Ltd.

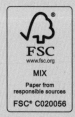

FSC
www.fsc.org
MIX
Paper from
responsible sources
FSC® C020056